SPORTSMASSAGE

Sportsmassage

by Jack Meagher & Pat Boughton

Illustrated by Pansy Haley

DOLPHIN BOOKS DOUBLEDAY & COMPANY, INC., Garden City, New York

Dolphin Books
Doubleday & Company, Inc.

Library of Congress Cataloging in Publication Data

Meagher, Jack.
  Sportsmassage.

  1. Massage.   2. Sports—Physiological aspects.
3. Physical fitness.   I. Boughton, Pat, joint author.
II. Title.
RC1226.M4   613.7'1
ISBN: 0-385-14556-X
Library of Congress Catalog Card Number 78–20085

To my wife, Betty Meagher, and our family, Jack, Kevin, Anne, Louise, Michelle, Bobby, Sean Michael, and Stacey,

and

To Ralph P. Hummel and my parents, Irene and Roy Boughton.

SPORTSMASSAGE: A PREFACE

The ancient Greeks had a saying for it: "Massage can never be fully appreciated by the common man."

This common man to whom they referred was not judged by wealth or social class. He was, rather, a man who lacked athletic grace. The athlete represented all the best characteristics of Greek culture. He was the man who willingly pushed himself time and again to the very limits of his endurance in order to achieve his goals. And even though he experienced pain with each maximum effort, he learned to live with it. He knew that his progress depended upon his ability to withstand that pain.

The same is true of the modern athlete. The pain of maximum effort is the hardest of all to withstand because unlike the pain of injury, it can be so easily stopped. All you have to do is *quit*. As steel is tempered in fire, so the athlete is developed by his courage and his determination to give to his sport everything he has to give. This was the ideal of the Greeks' "uncommon" man. This was—and is—the person who

can appreciate the benefits of Sportsmassage. While others may enjoy it, may use it for relaxation, or to relieve muscular problems, it is the athlete struggling to maintain his maximum effort who knows best the value of something that makes it a little bit easier, lets him go on a little farther, makes it possible for him to do a little bit better. Day by day.

In time, the concept of massage has changed. Because of its recognized ability to raise athletic performance levels, it was called upon to do the same in other areas where medical practice was still limited. Inevitably it failed more often than it succeeded. In the attempt to make massage work in this new surrounding, it was modified, changed, and partially emasculated. Its status today represents the divergence of the art of massage from its original purpose.

The most valuable contribution to the field of massage since the days of the Greeks was the percussion movements developed by the Swedish therapist Per Henrick Ling in the early part of this century. Known today as Swedish Massage, Ling's techniques quickly became very popular among Swedish cavalry officers as a relief from the exhaustion incurred from long hours on horseback. Though reminiscent of the powerful restorative techniques practiced by the Greeks, Swedish massage had one major drawback: It was performed at the end of the day after the body has suffered its quota of physical abuse. Thus there developed the irony that when proper massage was reintroduced into the sports world, it came as a restorative technique rather than as the protective, performance-boosting process of its original intent.

My Introduction to Sportsmassage

I was stationed in Europe immediately after World War II. I was NCO in charge of the camp dispensary at Epernay, France, and was playing football for the camp team. A German POW who performed various duties around the camp had been a masseur in Germany before the war. Whenever possible, he worked on me before a game. The difference this made in my ability to move while playing was astounding. It was especially interesting to me because although I had graduated from a school of Swedish Massage before going into the Army, I had never even heard of the kind of massage he was doing.

After my discharge, I went into professional baseball, signed by the Boston Braves as a pitcher. That career was short-lived, due to a wartime shoulder injury that recurred once I went into active training. The Braves did their best for me, trying all kinds of physical therapy, but a year later, I still could not throw a ball from the mound to home plate.

Then I went to a school of Viennese Massage in Connecticut run by another German instructor also familiar with the kind of massage I'd come to know in Europe. He found and relieved a few deeply seated muscular lesions in my chest, then more lesions at points on my shoulder far removed from the site of the actual pain. I learned to work on them myself and the shoulder improved so much that I was able to pitch semipro and town-team ball around Gloucester, Massachusetts, for another three years. What intrigued me most about the experience was that the specific areas used to alleviate my shoulder problem were *the exact same areas that the masseur in France used to concentrate on while preparing me for the game.* From that point on, I knew in what direction I wanted my work with massage to go. That was the beginning of what I now call *Sportsmassage.*

This book has been growing throughout my thirty-plus years' career in Sportsmassage. A lot of people have been helped by what I do and many of them have become as strong believers in it as I am. In fact, most of my clients—at least 90 per cent—are regulars who have been with me for years. One fellow is even such an enthusiast of Sportsmassage that he has willed his weekly appointment slot to his brother after he passes on himself.

A lot of these people have encouraged me to write this book. I'm glad for the way they feel about Sportsmassage, but sharing the techniques and the results is not the only reason I finally got down to putting this together. My interest is also in *why* Sportsmassage works, not simply that it does. So many years have gone into trying to find out the why and then proving it that it has become something like a passion with me. This book says some things that have never been said before in relation to massage. It explains some things that have never been explained before in relation to massage. And that is my real interest—to open up a new respect and respectability for my profession.

Everyone involved in this project is also a believer. Pat and Pansy speak for themselves below. But first I want to add my thanks to the fellows at the Salem and Malden YMCAs who repeatedly lent their strength and energy to the testings of Sportsmassage.

And a special thanks to William Johnson, M.D., orthopedic surgeon, for his help and support in preparing this book.

Jack Meagher
Lynn, Massachusetts
September 1978

Jack's right. I'm a believer too, and have been ever since my Uncle Ben started me out rubbing his back when I was a little girl. Since then I've been interested in both European and oriental massage techniques.

But I have never experienced anything like Sportsmassage. And I have never seen anything like the devotion of the athletes—professional and amateur—whom Jack works with.

Pat Boughton
Spruce Head Island, Maine
September 1978

Two years ago, a horse I was jumping plowed through a fence and fell, leaving me writhing in agony. When I woke up in the hospital I heard the phone ringing next to my bed, but when I reached out to answer it, my arms remained at my sides.

I was in tears, but I couldn't even reach for a Kleenex to dry them off. It was four months before I could brush my hair or bend my head far enough forward to buckle my belt.

This was two years ago. Last spring I was a member of a group who broke a record for the number of vertical feet skied from a helicopter in the Bugaboos in the Canadian Rockies.

That I could do it is largely due to the grace of God and to a man named Jack Meagher, who took me from the limbo where the doctors and therapists had left off and brought me back to a life of full physical activity.

A certain quantity of pain and immobility are a part of my daily life now. However, I am able to do my work and to enjoy strenuous exercise and the adventure of oceans and mountains and horses.

For that I am always grateful. And for that I am illustrating this book.

Pansy Haley
Pride's Crossing, Massachusetts
September 1978

CONTENTS

INTRODUCTION TO SPORTSMASSAGE:
THE 20 PER CENT EXTRA

Whatever sport you play, Sportsmassage will give you 20 per cent extra—extra performance, extra protection, extra time, per game, per season, per career. This means a lot to you whether you're a professional athlete who depends on bodily skill and power for your livelihood, a serious amateur, or even if you're mainly a Saturday quarterback athlete who plays a sport strictly for recreation. With Sportsmassage, you can do what you do better, longer, and more easily, raising your performance level at the same time that you lower the stress level it places on your body.

That seems hard for most people to believe until they've experienced it personally. Jim Nance, the great Boston Patriot fullback, felt the same way when he first heard about the kind of massage I was doing. But he was interested enough to give it a try anyway. At the time that we met, Jim was twenty-eight years old, an age when the years of physical punishment that football had subjected him to were beginning to have their effect on his legs. My

entire message to him consisted of the following two sentences:

"At what point in the game do your legs begin to tighten up and bother you?"

"Beginning of the fourth period," was the answer.

"I will guarantee you the entire game with absolutely no tightening."

We began using Sportsmassage and we never stopped, not as long as Jim Nance was with Boston. His evaluation was that it used to take him half an hour of exercise to get his legs loose before a ball game. "With this, they are loose when I reach the field and still loose two days later."

That was his 20 per cent extra of time and protection. In his performance, it showed up a little differently. After our first session together—fortunately it was before a practice game—Jim went out and played, he thought, the same as usual. But in fact, his timing was off. The increase in power and mobility he gained from the Sportsmassage treatment gave him that extra push so that he suddenly found himself beyond the hole before he made his cut. Too much of a good thing was the diagnosis. (This is true of most athletes who take up Sportsmassage after years of establishing a system of inner timing that corresponds with their power and speed.) Jim had to learn *to readjust his responses to deal with his higher performance level.*

Sportsmassage: The Benefits

Specifically, Sportsmassage can do five things for you:

1. Maintain your entire body in better physical condition.

2. Prevent injuries and loss of mobility in potential trouble spots.

3. Boost athletic performance and endurance.

4. Cure and restore mobility to injured muscle tissue.

5. Extend both the good health and the overall life of your athletic "career."

To give you a picture of the ability of Sportsmassage to increase mechanical efficiency, I'll describe a few of my early "test runs" with people I worked on at two YMCAs. Some of these men were good amateur athletes, and others were simply dedicated to the concept of exercise. Their ages ranged from 15 to 61 years. They all had one thing in common: They had all been at it for years. They had already established their performance records and were working against that standard, trying to improve on their best.

Test No. 1 was a swimmer, a man 61 years old, in excellent physical condition. He had been a New York City swimming champion in high school, and a member of the famous 1929 Columbia crew. A dedicated exercise man, he had maintained a daily swimming program ever since college. We tried Sportsmassage on February 21, and his time for a half-mile swim tested at 12 minutes, a drop from his usual 15. By June 16, with Sportsmassage he was down to a consistent average of 8:40 without any pushing, without any muscle tightening. When this man travels on business he keeps up his daily swim routine, but without the extra benefit of the massage, and his performance drops to 9:10 or 9:15—still quite an improvement from his original speed of 15 minutes.

Test No. 2 was a weight lifter, aged 17. Tested on 3 consecutive Fridays, his best bench press (before Sportsmassage) was 5 repetitions with 225 pounds. His best military press was 1 repetition with 120 pounds. Following Sportsmassage, he did 8 reps with 225 on bench and 2 reps with 130 on military press. On the second test, he added 5 pounds to every lift made during a 2-hour workout, and within 3 weeks he had jumped to 4 reps with 235 pounds on the bench press and increased 10 pounds on the incline press.

My third test was a 20-year-old runner who was a physical-education major and part-time YMCA director. At that point he had just finished his fastest mile—6:50. We began Sportsmassage techniques and his time dropped immediately to 6:33 with absolutely no fatigue. He went on to hold his speed at 6:36 without any massage for a period of time. Then we resumed Sportsmassage and he dropped and held it at 6:05.

Increased performance, reduced strain, longer athletic life—these are the benefits accrued by Sportsmassage for anyone willing to give it a test. For the professional athlete the results are even more dramatic. Dropping the body's natural resistance to forced movement—and professional athletes exist in a constant state of overextension of the muscular and nervous systems

—gives easier motion and extended playing time. It also lessens pain.

Reduction of Pain

Pain is the silent partner in the lives of the pros. You watch these fellows playing as if they don't have an ache in their bodies. Don't believe it: They all have *some* pain. Very recently I read an article in the newspaper, an interview with Rudolph Nureyev, which describes the situation better than I ever could:

Two hours after a performance when the body cools down, that's when the torture begins. Yes, it hurts every time. You go to bed with pain. When you wake up, you must measure your steps when you go to the loo because if you walk too fast, you may rupture something. But then hot baths, massage, revive you. Resuscitate you.

You always know what will happen next. Pain becomes familiar. You do some steps the day after a performance and your body is reacquainted with pain. That way there is no pain. Judging from the experience of Margot and myself, you cannot dance without pain. It is always there. It is foot, or it is toe, or it is knee, or it is ass. Or it is shoulder or it is God knows what. Always something is missing. You are never 100 per cent on stage. So you have to learn to dance with missing parts.

Always, *maximum effort is bodily abuse;* and the pain that results comes from trauma, injury that is occurring or that has already occurred to the affected muscle tissue. Permanent microdamage occurs each and every time you play in pain, and it will eventually have its effect as reduced mobility and a shortened athletic career.

Many athletes, like Nureyev, find massage a restorative factor that enables them to keep going. Still, it makes much more sense to use massage to *prevent the repeated damage before it happens.* They can do this by changing the type and timing of the therapy. This is the difference between traditional physical therapy or athletic training, and Sportsmassage.

Sportsmassage: The Goals

In developing the technique of Sportsmassage, I have set certain goals, all of which work toward the ideal of the perfect athlete. Not everyone achieves them 100 per cent across the board—but without variation, every man or woman who has worked with me in Sportsmassage has become clearly closer to realizing these goals than he or she would ever have thought possible. The goals behind Sportsmassage are to enable you to:

Achieve Total Movement

Achieve Total Power—and ward off occasional athletic "slumps"

Extend Your Athletic Life Span—and push back your athletic peak

Give You an Extra Chance—to reach your own personal goal

ACHIEVING TOTAL MOVEMENT

When a muscle tightens, it affects not only the group of muscles experiencing the spasm, but neighboring groups of muscles as well. The result is a rapid deterioration of both power and co-ordination. Two good examples of this can be found in baseball and boxing.

A batter awaiting the pitch holds the bat loosely, tightening his grip at the last instant before the swing. Were he to hold on tightly the entire time he waited for the pitch, the tension buildup would not only destroy the whiplike action of his wrists, but would also reduce the power of the entire arm.

A boxer holds his hands loosely until the last split second before throwing his punch. Tightly clenched fists drain the entire upper body region in an amazingly short time. Try it for yourself. Make rapid arm movements holding your fists loosely clenched. Then do it again with them clenched tight. See how much more quickly you feel the strain in your upper arms. Undue tension and tightening in *any* part of the body reduce the effectiveness of the entire body.

I still can't think of a greater living example of the concept of Total Movement than Muhammad Ali—the speed, the ease with which he moves, the force he generates with a simple flick of the arm and wrist. As simple as he makes it look, he has the ability to place his entire body in the service of his fists so that what seems to the observer to be a flicking jab is in reality a solid blow that will snap an opponent's head back.

Making Muscles Work Toward Total Movement

A muscle can never be neutral—if it doesn't work for you, it works against you. Actively. A few fiber blocks scattered throughout the body, even those so minimal you are not aware of their existence, can interfere with the overall kinetic timing, the perfect synchronization that must occur in athletics in order to have co-ordination and freedom of movement.

A muscle problem is basically nothing more than an exaggeration of a normal condition—the contraction of a muscle. When, for various reasons, the contraction fails to release, it becomes a spasm, a rigid knot. The only difference between one muscle problem and another, short of an actual tearing of the tissue, is the extent of the spasm and its location. Even a muscle tear, once the breach has been healed, has the same basic physiology.

Now, rest can help to work out a simple kink or spasm, but once the problem has developed into a deep-seated lesion, you're living in a fool's paradise if you think that simply laying off for a while will do the trick. Lesions develop as the result of a trauma to a muscle region, accompanied by inflammation. The inflammation produces edema, thick fluid the body secretes as a healing agent—what you find when you break a blister.

The side effect is that this liquid acts like a mild form of cement, binding the tissue fibers together in an adhesion. So you now have fibers in spasm with reduced blood and oxygen supply—a cause of spasm—being rendered immovable by the cementing action of the edema. You may overcome the symptoms with pain killers and muscle relaxants, but you won't get rid of the spasm. You may go on and return to your sport, but you will only aggravate the lesion and develop stress and strain at some other point in your body.

Sportsmassage *before* the spasms reach the critical stage is the only sensible way to keep your entire muscular structure in top form. This is a new way of thinking for most people, who see massage mainly in terms of correcting known problems. *Sportsmassage provides the two physiological ingredients necessary for re-establishing complete muscular function: massage and exercise.* It moves individual muscle fibers in imitation of their normal motion. It establishes hyperemia, an extra supply of blood and oxygen, where it is most critically needed. The hyperemia produced by Sportsmassage lasts for several hours, long enough to allow a deep muscle prob-

SPORTSMASSAGE

xvii

lem to relax and respond to follow-up exercises. Or, in optimum conditions, the effects of Sportsmassage can last long enough to allow you to complete an entire athletic event with full power and fluidity. The basis behind loosening up of fibers and the establishment of hyperemia is the same whether it is applied to your entire body before competition or to a single trouble-causing spot. It prepares the muscle to function at its peak mechanical efficiency—to achieve Total Movement.

ACHIEVING TOTAL POWER

Full, powerful motion is in actuality a synchronized wave of smaller motions rather than a single, simultaneous movement. Whatever move you make in whatever sport you play, a series of successive muscle groups are brought into action, one by one. Each feeds upon and magnifies the force and motion generated by the preceding muscle groups, to the point that the ultimate motion is in fact more powerful than the sum total of the individual movements.

For example, take the complete motion of pitching a baseball. The solid base is the sole of the foot on the side of the throwing arm. The opposite arm and leg act as counterbalance for a backward motion used to gain the fullest possible sweep. From this back point, all motion must be directed forward at the target.

In this forward sweep there are three distinct, co-ordinated movements that start with the lower body in the stride, continue with the trunk—using the pelvis as its solid base—twisting and bending in the direction of the target, and finish off with the shoulder, arm, and hand coming forward in that order. The final projection of the ball off the fingers is the culmination of

what began at the sole of the foot. Regardless of sidearm or overhand delivery, the order of movement must be the same, the only difference being the amount of torso twist as the trunk is flexed.

Power loss is easier to spot than Total Power. You can recognize power loss a mile off. Watch a local Little League or high-school baseball game, and you're sure to see at least one youngster out there pitching with improper technique and follow-through. Usually you'll see his shoulder and arm begin their sweep ahead of or simultaneously with the trunk. If the torso is ahead of the legs, it works against the power generated by them. If the arm is ahead of the torso, it nullifies the power created by it. Regardless of how strong the pitcher is or how hard he tries, until he falls into the proper sequence of motion, he has no fast ball.

Total Power is the end result of co-ordinated Total Movement. Total Power is not the same thing as strength. *Strength is a contractive function* on the part of a muscle. This is fine by itself, but try walking around with contracted muscles, and all you're likely to get out of it is a cramp. Co-ordination and *power depend on the ability of a muscle to relax* as well as to contract.

If you have trouble drawing this fine line of distinction between pure strength and Total Power, consider for a moment the case of the power weight lifter vs. the Olympic weight lifter. Though considered primarily a question of strength, successful weight lifting—as well as most other sports—relies upon the utilization of the three basic units of motion described earlier in regard to the baseball pitcher. Legs. Torso. Shoulders and arms. While in all instances, the three movements follow each other so closely they appear simultaneous, the main application of each is slightly behind the others in timing, particularly in power lifting. Power lifting is in fact misnamed: It is pure strength. Its three lifts—the bench press, the squat, and the dead lift—do not require the co-ordinated motion needed to get the weight overhead as in Olympic lifting. I have known and worked with superb class power lifters with tremendous strength who have attempted Olympic-style lifting in contests only to finish well behind Olympic-trained men with less strength primarily because they could not achieve that one, two, three co-ordination of contraction and relaxation necessary to "get under the bar" at shoulder level.

Sportsmassage facilitates Total Power by preparing the body to deliver a harmonious flow of energy and force from one area to another. The condition of hyperemia that gives you Total Movement keeps the channels of your internal system open and "go" so you can pull off the necessary power punch when the game calls for it.

Sportsmassage and Athletic Slumps

Athletic slumps seem to be an accepted part of the athletic life: Everyone is sorry, but most take it in stride that a crack ball pitcher, for instance, can go from being a nine-inning worker to one who can't last beyond the fourth or the fifth. What happens? He hasn't lost his strength. He hasn't lost his ability. He has lost, through a degree of residual muscle tightening, that ultimate co-ordination that made him what he was.

Uusually when this happens an athlete is "sat down" for a period of time until he loosens up to where he can regain his potential. It works okay, most of the time. But underneath in a majority of cases, a loss occurs. It may be a loss of time which can be crucial in terms of a player's overall record in a highly competitive field. Or it

may be a loss of overall range of power dealt by the development of muscle spasms overlooked because no actual pain was present. These are the saddest cases because these athletes never fully regain their lost form and never find out why. For them, the big game is over.

Sportsmassage finds the spasm and works it out. Sportsmassage keeps the athlete's body in prime working condition even while he is sidelined or on the bench. Sportsmassage sends him back into the game with full power.

INCREASING YOUR ATHLETIC LIFE SPAN

Nothing lasts forever. Your body can be likened to your car in some respects. It ages and the more hard miles you put on it, the faster wear and tear show up. With proper care and maintenance, it lasts longer and gives you better performance along the way. The big difference is that when your car reaches the point of no return, you can trade it in on another.

Being born with a healthy body is largely a matter of God's good grace. Maintaining its functioning abilities is up to you. Your body represents everything you have done to it and for it. The day that you cannot do what you were able to do yesterday, you have gone backward. Your first slippage will be a direct result of accumulated mileage and injuries.

Slippage will occur in three stages:

1. You will be able to do everything you have been doing, but it will become exhausting rather than tiring. It will take a longer time to recuperate between sessions.

2. You will be able to do everything you have been doing, but for shorter periods of time.

3. You can't do it.

This last instance is inevitable, but the space between No. 1 and No. 3 can be prolonged considerably by proper training and proper living habits. It is the untreated development of muscle tightening early on, either in a game or in a career, that increases the body's resistance to full, fluid movement. In turn, it increases the amount of energy you have to put out to maintain a top pace, and reduces the time this pace can be maintained.

The prominent cause of diminishing abilities in the healthy athletic body, no matter what the age, is the buildup of years of microtrauma associated with maximum effort combined with the results of old, unresolved injuries. Where Sportsmassage has been used over the years to lessen the trauma and maintain pliability of muscle tissue, joint flexibility, and to more fully restore full motion following injury, this buildup will not be so great nor come so soon.

Sportsmassage and the Beginning Athlete

Case: A person middle-aged or older with a high-stress, low-activity job goes to the doctor. Diagnosis: overweight, high blood pressure. Prognosis: a physical breakdown, a stroke, or a heart attack.

Whereas forty years ago, the prescription would have been complete rest or an ocean voyage, today it is exercise. A series of short walks is usually the physician's first recommendation, but in truth it takes much more to rebuild good body tone. The benefit derived from exercise will be in direct correlation to the amount performed: *The two worst things for the muscular system are overuse and no use.* Somewhere in between, in graduated amounts, is the right use.

Sportsmassage introduced into your rehabilitation program at this point will allow you to do X amount of exercise with 20 per cent less exhaustion, while reducing the possibility of myositis or overuse and strain. Most important in this situation is that the massage be carried out *before* the exercise is done.

Moving Back Your Athletic Peak

Let's return to the case of the totally healthy athlete. No matter what the sport, any runner, swimmer, weight lifter, and so forth can tell you about the barrier that develops as you near your peak. When you first begin a sport, improvement comes rapidly; and increased teaching, technique, and practice bring even more gains. However, eventually you will come to the point where progress is painfully slow or nonexistent. What has happened is that you have reached your athletic peak; physically, your muscles are tightening, resisting maximum effort.

Sportsmassage can move back that barrier. It makes sense. Instead of forcing yourself to push, push, push against the wall, why not reach around behind it and move it back?

GIVING YOURSELF AN EXTRA CHANCE

As the song says, most of us "only go around once." If you do somehow get the opportunity to give it one more whirl, Sportsmassage can make the difference that changes your personal history. I know that sounds dramatic, but it can happen. And it has. I've seen it.

"A thirty-two-year-old professional football player recently came to me with a hamstring and a calf pull that were threatening to close out his season prematurely. This man was a defensive lineman, who in his younger days had been at three different NFL training camps, but had been released for lack of quickness. There was no problem with his strength, determination, and love of vigorous combat.

But he just hadn't made the big time. This last year, however, he got his extra chance, and he credits Sportsmassage with the honors. As a result of our work, he picked up time to the point where he was just named "defensive lineman of the year" for the second year running. And his new-found speed has earned him an invitation to an NFL team for this coming season. In his own words, "I'm five yards quicker than I ever was."

Everything about Sportsmassage is an "extra." It is the practical application of kinesiology that provides extra help for motion problems beyond the scope of physical therapy. It is a counterbalance to the effects of strain and overexertion, which means an extra measure of protection and performance unattainable by training and conditioning alone.

And its most important "extra" is time . . . time to do what *you* want to do at the level at which *you* want to do it!

HOW TO USE THIS BOOK

There are three ways to use this book. That is, there are three sections that tell you how to do your own Sportsmassage, depending on your specific goals.

First, you can use Sportsmassage in its entirety, following the description of the Total Body Massage in the appropriate chapter, "How to Do It."

Second, you can use Sportsmassage *directed at your particular sport* and its most common problems, following the descriptions in the *chapters on the individual sports in Part Two* of the book.

Third, you can use Sportsmassage *directed at particular problems,* following the descriptions for individual trouble spots in the "On the Spot" chapter at the end of the book.

Part One

How It Works

To know the basis of Sportsmassage is to learn the names of the major muscles, the bones for which they provide movement, and the direction of that movement. This entails the study of osteology and myology, which most of you probably will not want to go into too deeply at this point. Therefore this section, called "Basic Body Mechanics," will provide you with the practical information you need to practice Sportsmassage on your own.

THE SKELETAL SYSTEM—HOW IT WORKS

Osteology is the study of the skeleton, the support foundation of the body. It consists of two hundred bones of four different classifications:

1. *Long bones,* the levers for action—the arms and legs;

2. *Flat bones,* designed to present sufficient surface area for the attachment of the heavy trunk muscles—the sternum (breastbone), scapula (shoulder blade), pelvis; these bones are largely immobile

and provide the solid base for the leverlike action of the limbs;

3. *Short bones,* found mainly in the ankles and feet and spaced to cushion the shock of concussion; the patella (kneecap) is usually included in this classification;

4. *Irregular bones,* the vertebrae and bones of the skull and face.

Muscles are attached to bones by sheets of tendonous tissue stretched onto the rounded ends of the bones and the rough, irregular surfaces along the shafts.

The union of two or more bones or cartilage is called an articulation or *joint.* The immovable joints, such as those of the skull or pelvis, are not the concern of Sportsmassage. The movable joints are the points where skeletal, and thus body, motion take place.

The ends of these movable bones are held in place by ligaments and joint capsules. *Ligaments* are strong, fibrous bands, some interwoven into the joint capsule. Others form extra, heavier lateral and medial support. These are called *collateral ligaments* and are a frequent source of joint problems that can be dealt with very successfully with Sportsmassage. *Cartilage* is interspaced between the ends of bones as shock absorbers. It cannot be treated by massage.

HOW MUSCLES WORK

Myology is the study of muscles, their attachments to bones, and the action they provide.

The skeletal muscles are called striated or striped muscles. They are *voluntary muscles,* functioning upon command. Example: You bend or straighten your arm when you wish to do so.

Another classification is the nonstriated or smooth muscles—the *involuntary muscles.* These function without conscious effort on your part as the muscles involving respiration, intestinal peristalsis, etc. The heart muscles, while striated, are also involuntary and so fall into a separate classification.

Muscles have two ends. A fixed attachment called the *origin*—usually closer to the midline of the body—and the movable attachment called the *insertion.*

The thickened middle of the muscle is called the *belly.* It is at this point that the motor nerve enters the muscle and produces nerve impulses that stimulate contraction. The initial contraction of fibers takes place here, then spreads to the end of the muscle as greater contraction is needed to accomplish a given task.

Each fiber has its own nerve supply so that it can be stimulated without affecting its neighbors—the "All-or-none Response." While in a relaxed state, each fiber is like a soft thread. When contracted, it has enough force to support a thousand times its own weight. But without a nerve impulse, there can be no contraction.

The speed with which a muscle contracts depends a great deal upon its viscosity—the thickness of individual fibers. Thin muscles have less resistance, therefore contract and recover faster. Speed, such as sprinting, is usually associated with low-viscosity muscles; strength, then, with those of high viscosity. This is why *different types of muscle are better suited to different types of activity.*

It is important to keep in mind that a body is born with a fixed number of muscle fibers. You can never add to that number. Increase in muscle size comes not from added fibers, but from the thickening of those that already exist.

When muscle fibers are lost through *atrophy* you can never get them back. Disease is a cause of atrophy. So is injury. So is disuse; which makes it imperative that you find a way to maintain activity as soon as possible following any sort of physical disablement.

Forceful muscle activity causes the fibers to enlarge—*hypertrophy.* It increases both the motive power of the muscle and the nutrient mechanism that maintains that increased power. Hypertrophy results mainly from extremely forceful working of the muscles even though the activity might occur for only a few minutes each day. At least 75 per cent of a muscle's strength is required to build hypertrophy. This is the reason *strength can be developed in muscles more rapidly when resistive or isometric exercise is used rather than simple, prolonged mild exercise.*

The Facts of Fat

Muscles are of necessity a vascular tissue. Fat is a nonvascular tissue, having no network of blood vessels of its own. Its presence in, between, and around muscle fibers increases resistance to motion, the blood and oxygen supply, and reduces the ability of muscles to perform their functions. Fat is a noncontractile tissue. Even a hundred pounds of fat cannot lift one ounce of weight one inch!

Oxygen—The Indispensable Factor

Oxygen is the fuel of combustion in muscular activity. Adequate oxygen delivery depends on many factors: inspired oxygen concentration, the pulmonary system, heart, lungs, blood vessels, and the microcirculation with which Sportsmassage is most concerned. It is at this point that the oxygen-carrying portion of the blood must leave the vessels, filter through the tissues to deposit nutrient, pick up by-products of combustion, and be reabsorbed into the venous system. This is the weak link in the circulatory chain. It is the "combat zone" where everything happens—or doesn't happen! It is not superficial. It is the necessary link in the deepest part of your muscular structure. It is the point where Sportsmassage gives that extra boost.

Insufficient oxygen and the accumulation of lactic acid, a by-product of combustion, cause muscles to weaken. Lactic acid is produced by metabolism when an insufficient amount of oxygen is present—*anoxia.* Lactic acid levels rise in direct proportion to the lack of oxygen, causing the muscle to lose its ability for complete performance.

From the time it leaves the heart, blood is forced through ever-narrowing channels —arteries, arterioles, and finally into a vast network of minute blood vessels called *capillaries.* The walls of the capillaries are dotted with permeable areas called stomata through which the oxygen-charged portion of the blood is discharged into the tissues.

In muscles, the shape of the capillary network is elongated to run parallel to the long axis of the fibers. The number and size of the capillaries and the interspace between them are determining factors as to how much oxygenated blood can be delivered to and how much metabolic waste can be discharged from any given area. *This is the vital feeding and cleansing process for which your entire circulatory system is structured.*

The meshes and interspaces are much wider apart in ligamentous tissue, fascia, and fibers of lesser use than in the belly of the muscle. Therefore, the musculotendonous junction has a five or six to one ratio for primary breakdown as well as for the development of a spasm due to anoxia and lactic acid formation during strenuous activity.

Richness is where muscle action is. Richness is not where the stress overload takes place! It is the combination of these two factors that is manifested as stress points in the body. Any pre-existing degree of tightening or spasm that causes fibers to lie more closely or rigidly together further

SPORTSMASSAGE APPLIED TO MUSCLE SPASM
EFFECTS OF HYPEREMIA

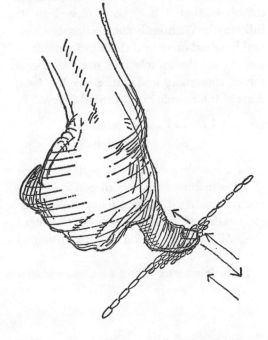

hinders the free flow of oxygen into and the removal of toxins from the muscle.

Training and conditioning of course increase the ability of the heart and lungs to oxygenate and pump blood and of the muscles to produce work. *The fiber-spreading technique of Sportsmassage—by creating a durable hyperemia that enlarges the capillaries and increases the interspace and by rendering tissue fibers more pliable—increases even more the ability of the muscle to receive and utilize fuel and efficiently cast off toxins.*

How Muscles Move—Contraction and Relaxation

To understand this concept, you have to really understand the meaning of relaxation. If you think of it as a lethargic, sleepy state such as lying in a sauna or on a sunny beach, you're missing the point. *Relaxation is a lack of restrictive tension* that allows unimpaired movement in any direction. In the specific case of Sportsmassage, it is a release of tension.

Muscles generate motion. They also restrict motion. Muscles are arranged in pairs of opposites, and a muscle does two things: It contracts, and between contractions it relaxes so that it may be stretched to its full length. With each contraction the several hundred or several thousand *myofibrils* making up the muscle fold over on themselves, shortening and thickening the total mass of the muscle as illustrated below.

- - - - - - - -   relaxation
    z   contraction

As a muscle contracts, it pulls the bone of its attachment in the direction of the contraction. As it relaxes, its opposite muscle is allowed to pull the bone the other way. All skeletal motion is a repetition of this basic process.

There is no such thing as a muscle that pushes. *All muscles pull.* The pulling of certain muscle groups may produce a pushing action by the body against an outside object. But the muscles in themselves give motion through the shortening action.

In this alternate contraction and relaxation process, you find the fundamental difference between strength and power. *Strength comes from the size of a muscle plus its ability to contract. Power is the degree of movement that this contraction achieves.* If the relaxing muscle does not stretch to its fullest extent, or is slow to stretch, you have increased resistance, reduced power, and therefore reduced performance levels.

Everyone is familiar with the case of the "muscle-bound" person who possesses fantastic strength but can be outdone by someone with *less strength but greater power.* The same principle applies, in a much lesser degree, to a muscle that must undergo the rigors and repeated microtrauma of training and competition.

Any muscle that is consistently worked within the same range of motion will shorten as it gains strength. To protect himself against this shortening, the human athlete employs a daily routine of stretching exercises designed to extend muscles to their fullest. If he doesn't do this, his performance levels drop along with his mobility and resistance and he becomes prone to serious muscle injuries.

The Fragility of Overtight Muscles

Muscle tightening can cause weakening and danger. During any sustained activity, the intake of oxygen and the concurrent removal of waste products become insufficient for the needs of the muscle. *Because the contraction process is a generated action and the relaxation process is not, it is the latter process that is the first to deteriorate.*

When this happens, muscles do not stretch as completely or as quickly, and the contractors are forced to work harder to overcome the increased resistance. Result: both a loss of power and an increase in energy output necessary to maintain the same pace.

This you see as "the fade." Labored motion, dull reflexes, shortened range of movement. The lead into this has begun, of course, long before "the fade." It began with the very first step. *The final stage of muscle tightening is muscle fatigue—the complete loss of power.*

Muscle tightening and muscle fatigue are the natural results of maximum effort. They are inevitable but not unalterable! My work with athletes at two YMCAs has proven a consistent 20 per cent improvement in the maintenance of peak muscle function following the application of Sportsmassage. Not only will you start loose and stay loose, you will also have fewer problems along the way to a full and maximum performance.

The "All-or-none Response"

Mentioned earlier, the "All-or-none Response" is a major factor in muscle problems. What it basically amounts to is the straightforward fact that you cannot use an entire muscle "a little bit!" Muscles are arranged in bundles of fibers, each acting independently of its neighbors, and only the number of fibers required to perform an action are brought into play.

Fibers either contract to their fullest or do not contract at all. Maximum effort brings fibers into play that do not ordinarily get use. Fibers situated at the ends of the muscle have less elasticity. This renders them more susceptible to each successive strain and overexertion. It also allows these spasms to go unnoticed until they reach the critical stage of causing dis-

comfort, pain, or disablement. And once that has occurred, it renders them much more difficult to treat by massage.

This explains why, no matter how well conditioned you are, you develop problems following a particular grueling session of sports playing. A proper warmup is naturally essential. But is is not enough to reach all of the muscular structure you will use during such a session. A warmup is not a loosening or a stretching process. A warmup is a raising of the temperature of muscles to their proper operating levels. It does not eliminate existing spasms, it overcomes them.

Sportsmassage before the event assures that the fibers of least use in every muscle to be used can receive proper attention and protection. Without it, you risk postplay charley horse and, even more troublesome, the perplexing kind of muscle problem that drags on and on for months for seemingly no reason at all.

Muscle Fatigue—The End of the Line

Prolonged and sharp contraction of a muscle leads to the well-known state of muscle fatigue associated with a loss of power. It results simply from the inability of the contractile and metabolic processes of the muscle fibers to continue supplying the level of work output. The nerve continues to work normally. The impulses pass normally through the neuromuscular junction into the muscle fiber. Normal action potential spreads over the fiber but the contraction becomes weaker as the nutrient source is downcut.

Interruption of blood supply to a fiber causes complete loss of power in one minute's time because the oxidation of glucose, the body's main energy supply, cannot take place. The same situation occurs when intense effort or prolonged exertion has used fuel and oxygen faster than it could be supplied to the muscle tissue. At this point, the body shifts gears into a process called *glycolysis,* a type of alternate energy system that is better than nothing but nowhere near as effective as oxidation.

The scientific Law of Mass Action states that as the end products of a chemical reaction build up in the reacting medium, the rate of the reaction approaches zero. In plain words, you have to get rid of the ashes to make room for the coal or the fire goes out.

In the case of glycolysis, the ashes or end products convert to lactic acid ultimately, which in turn is absorbed by other cells of less active use, thereby spreading the fatigue over a wider area—a last-ditch effort of sorts to prevent the total breakdown of the individually overworked portion of the body.

Once the contest is over, you repay the oxygen debt to the overexerted parts of the body by the heavy breathing that continues on after the exertion itself is ended. The chemical process, enriched once more by the presence of sufficient oxygen, reverses itself: Lactic acid breaks down into the component parts that convert themselves back into glucose, and the condition stabilizes. The overall impression is one of the body as a self-rechargeable battery.

While the type of ultimate breakdown we have been discussing here is generally associated with endurance sports such as distance running or swimming, it is also a familiar phenomenon for athletes in training. Pushing yourself to this degree is a necessary part of muscle development and athletic ability. You push for your maximum. The longer you can go before reaching it, the more you can do. The more you can do, the better you get.

For a full explanation of the physiology discussed in brief here, see the Appendix at the end of the book.

THE BASIC MECHANICS OF SPORTSMASSAGE

All massage brings blood and oxygen to muscles. That is a plus, but one that is soon used up. The deep and repetitive compressions of the fiber-spreading techniques of Sportsmassage produce a *hyperemia,* not just a milking of the tissues. The method of compression extends the hyperemia—a dilation of the total range of blood vessels—along the full depth and extent of the muscle.

Hyperemia is maintained by the presence of histamines and acetylcholine, which the repeated in-depth compressions release. *Muscle fibers are thoroughly worked out, repeatedly spread apart to increase their pliability in expanding and contracting, shortening and broadening.* Along the way, the numerous tiny spasms that resist stretching are relieved and specific areas of stress overload receive the extra push needed to get them through the contest ahead.

One after another the "extras" pay off. . . . An increase in free motion is achieved because of increased pliability. . . . Free motion is maintained because a pliable muscle more readily responds to demands to contract and relax. . . . Hyperemia increases the vital supply of oxygen and maintains efficient removal of waste matter, and in doing so pushes back the time when anoxia and toxic buildup force glycolysis to take over the system.

The free motion established with Sportsmassage is conserving your energy with each and every body movement you make from start to finish.

BASIC MOVEMENTS AND STRESS POINTS

Every body has mechanical weaknesses. These weaknesses occur where stress overload is greatest as the body performs certain movements. The relationship between such stress points and basic movements forms the crux of Sportsmassage. Understanding that relationship tells you where to expect trouble, when it's most likely, and what to do about it.

Whatever sport you play, whatever position you play in that sport, and however good you are at it, you operate within the framework of one or more of twelve basic movements. Each sport employs a certain variety of these movements and when you go through the motions of using them, you tax certain related stress points on your body. These are the first areas to break down during sustained effort and the last to recover: They are the lead-in for all muscle tightening, muscle fatigue, loss of mobility or power, and slowing down of reflexes and co-ordination.

The following pages illustrate the twelve basic movements and the stress points inherent in each. Learn to identify the basic movements connected with your sport. And learn to check yourself out for the particular stress points taxed by that sport. Once you learn these basic facts of your athletic life, you can maintain a more or less constant reading of your Total Movement quotient. And you can give yourself an instant boost whenever and wherever it's needed.

BASIC MOVEMENT NO. 1—*Deep Knee Bend*

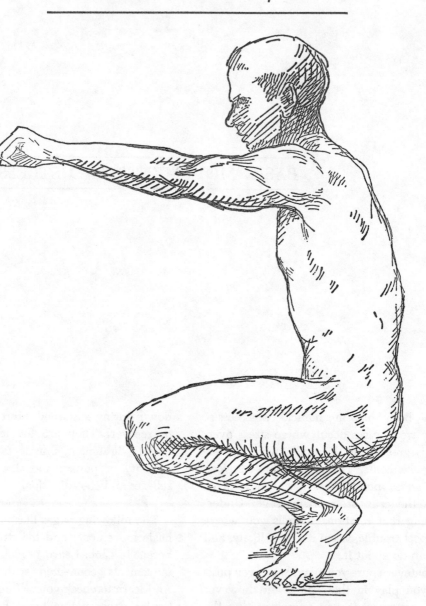

Maximum-stress Areas	*Maximum-stress Sports*
Lower back	Cycling
Buttocks	Dancing
Hips	Football
Thighs, front and back	Skating
	Skiing
	Tennis
	Weight lifting

BASIC MOVEMENT NO. 2—*Leg-forward Stretch*

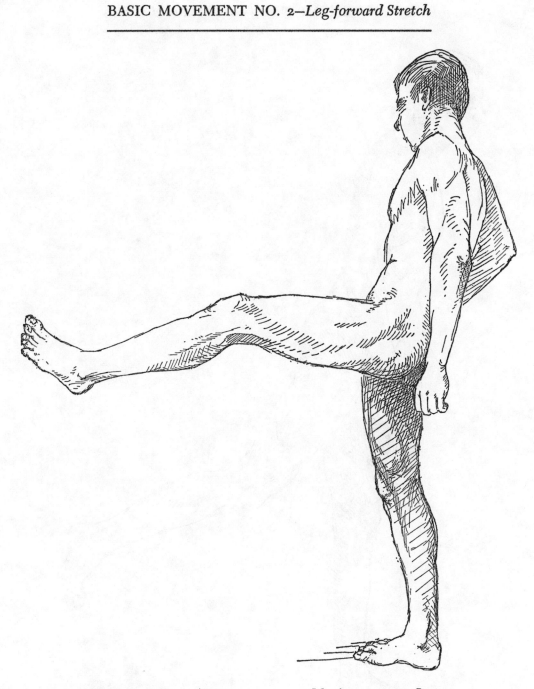

Maximum-stress Areas

Upper hamstring, thigh
Outer calf

Maximum-stress Sports

Basketball
Dancing
Football
Skating

BASIC MOVEMENT NO. 3—*Leg-backward Stretch*

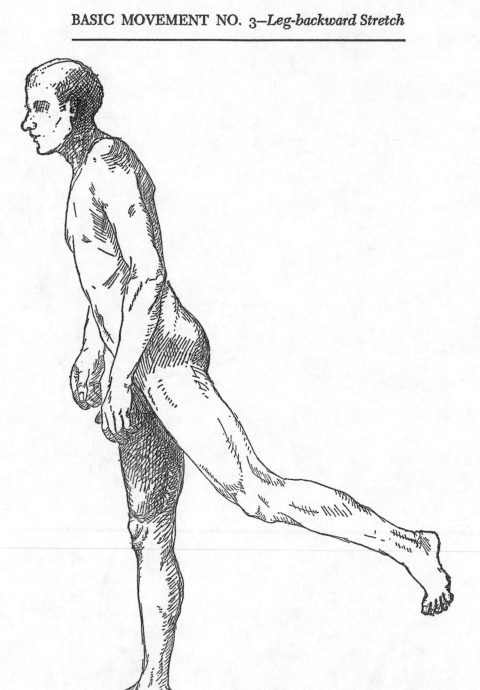

Maximum-stress Areas

Groin
Front hip
Abdomen
Thigh, front

Maximum-stress Sports

Hockey
Skating

BASIC MOVEMENT NO. 4—*Leg-sideways Stretch*

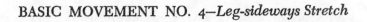

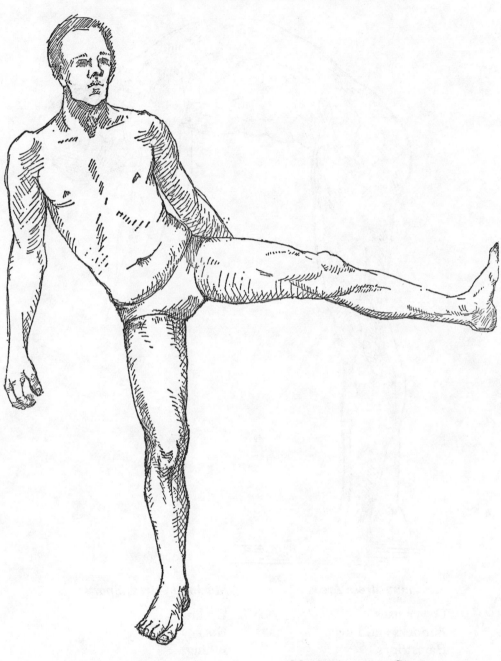

Maximum-stress Areas

Groin
Inner thigh

Maximum-stress Sports

Riding
Soccer

BASIC MOVEMENT NO. 5—*Trunk-forward Bend*

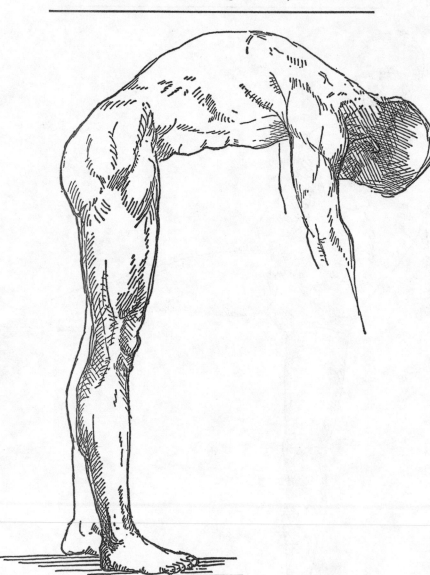

Maximum-stress Areas

Lower back
Buttocks and hips
Hamstrings
Back of knees, calves

Maximum-stress Sports

Cycling
Hockey
Riding
Skating
Tennis

BASIC MOVEMENT NO. 6—*Trunk-backward Bend*

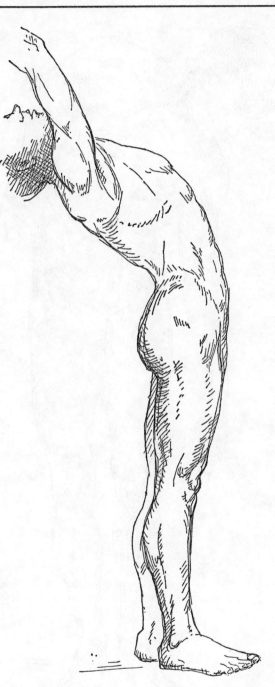

Maximum-stress Areas	*Maximum-stress Sports*
Abdomen	Dancing
Hips, front	Tennis
Thighs, front	

BASIC MOVEMENT NO. 7—*Trunk-side Bend*

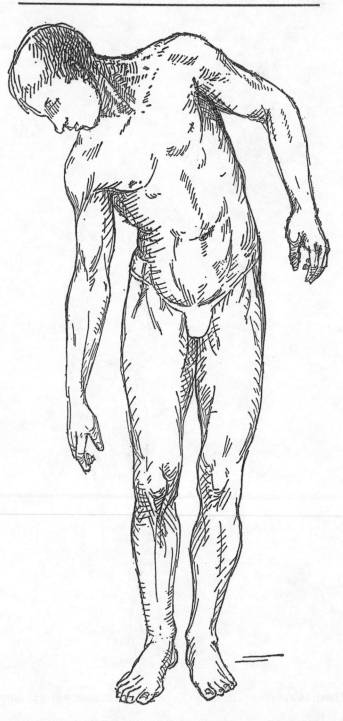

Maximum-stress Areas

Waist
Hips
Outside legs to midcalf

Maximum-stress Sports

Body building
Weight lifting

BASIC MOVEMENT NO. 8—*Trunk Twist*

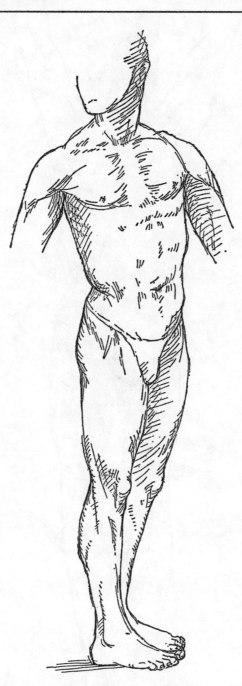

Maximum-stress Areas	*Maximum-stress Sports*
Hips	Body building
Lower back	Dancing
Abdomen	Golf
Front of groin	Soccer
Knees, side of thighs	Tennis
	Weight lifting

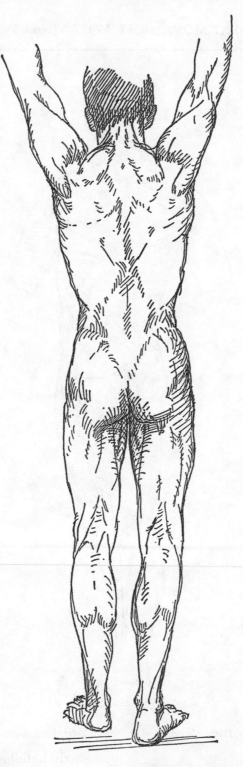

Maximum-stress Areas

Back of arm
Side of trunk
Upper back, midback

Maximum-stress Sports

Basketball
Swimming

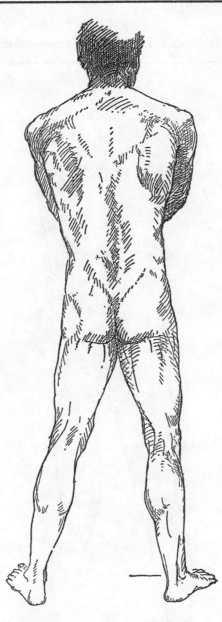

Maximum-stress Areas

Arms, front and side
Neck, front and back
Shoulder blade

Maximum-stress Sports

Cycling
Golf
Hockey
Riding
Swimming

BASIC MOVEMENT NO. 11—*Arms-backward Stretch*

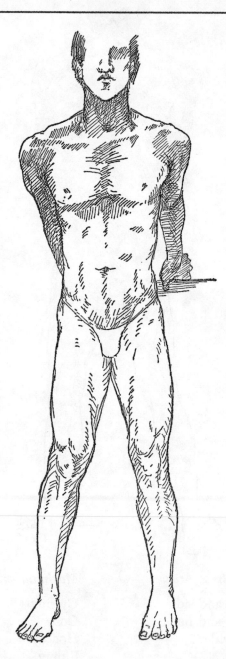

Maximum-stress Areas

Arms, back and sides

Maximum-stress Sport

Tennis

BASIC MOVEMENT NO. 12—*Arms-downward Stretch*

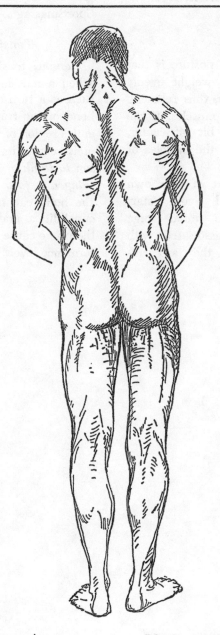

Maximum-stress Areas	*Maximum-stress Sports*
Shoulders	Dancing
Arms	Swimming
Neck	Weight lifting

THE POSTURE AND EXERCISE CONNECTION

The importance of good posture is that the erect body places its weight evenly upon the skeletal structure, thus relieving the constant strain on the muscles. If the head is carried the least bit off center, more tension is applied to the muscles of the neck.

You may never be aware of your own posture problems until you start Sportsmassage—for in the initial stage there are no symptoms associated with these posture points until they are subjected to the manual pressure of Sportsmassage.

Tension and Exercise

Nervous tension tightens muscles. And when a muscle is tight, a simple motion such as a turn of the head, a sneeze, or a bend of the trunk is enough to spasm an entire region of the body. This is where exercise comes in. *It is impossible for a person to think of many problems while pursuing any form of vigorous exercise.* But the body can only do what is within its capabilities, and muscle tightening is still the prime cause of reduced power and performance levels.

THE ART

Sportsmassage is hard work! The recipient can only get out of it what you put into it. You are, in a manner of speaking, adding your strength to his. At your fingertips you have—once you learn to use it—the most powerful of all the therapeutic modalities. The granddaddy of them all! *Every piece of physical-therapy equipment—from the most elaborate and expensive right down to the simple hot compress—is an attempt to produce the results of Sportsmassage— hyperemia and therapeutic movement.*

The most important thing to achieve with Sportsmassage is depth, and because every body is different every body possesses a different tolerance to pressure. Different parts of the body, even the same body, have varied tolerances. While the breaking up of the spasms is painful, the general massage is never so. It is forceful, not brutal. Reaction of the player is your best guide. If he shows discomfort, or tightens up under your hands, either your pressure is too great or your technique is faulty. You seek to release tightening, not to cause it.

Do not associate depth with pain and do not cater to masochistic tendencies. A surprising number of people *want* a massage to hurt and are not satisfied unless they are forced to grit their teeth. Of course, some people simply lack surface sensitivity. A man with a hide like an elephant will want a massage like an elephant.

To apply great force without causing discomfort, pain, or unwanted symptoms is a goodly part of the art of Sportsmassage. And it is what should be practiced. It is the part that the onlooker cannot see or understand. The results must be experienced before understanding is possible.

THE STROKES

There are four basic, therapeutic strokes in Sportsmassage: *direct pressure, friction, compression,* and *percussion.* Two more— *effleurage* and *kneading*—are supplementary strokes used in conjunction with the four basic ones when the occasion calls for it.

The pressing action that forms the basis

of all Sportsmassage movements can be applied with the palm of the hand, the loose fist, the heel of the hand, the pads of the fingers, or the points of the fingers. Look at the accompanying illustrations closely and you notice that in each successive movement you are concentrating the pressure you apply upon a smaller and smaller area, thus gaining greater penetration and depth. The direction, or thrust, of the force you use is always inward—down into and spreading out through the muscle.

DIRECT PRESSURE

Direct pressure is self-explanatory. You push in with a fingertip, thumb, or braced finger—straight in—and hold the press for fifteen to sixty seconds, depending upon the situation. This is the take-off point of Sportsmassage and the premier stroke with which you approach virtually all stress points on the body.

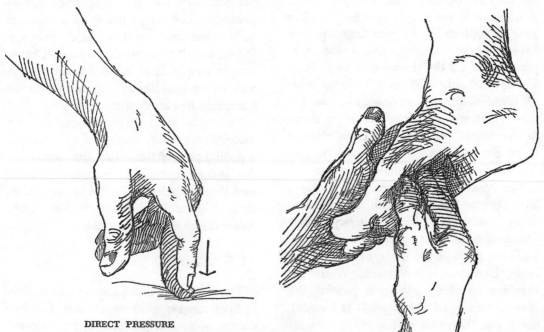

DIRECT PRESSURE
BRACED FINGER

DIRECT PRESSURE
TIPS OF FINGERS

FRICTION

Friction is a stroke that is a direct offshoot of *direct pressure*. Applied with a fingertip, thumb, braced finger, fist, or palm of the hand, the stroke is the basic push in and hold with an added component of movement. Move your fingers to and fro and you have crossfiber *friction*. Move them around in a small circle and you have circular *friction*.

Friction and *direct pressure* are the basic one-two sequence used in Sportsmassage.

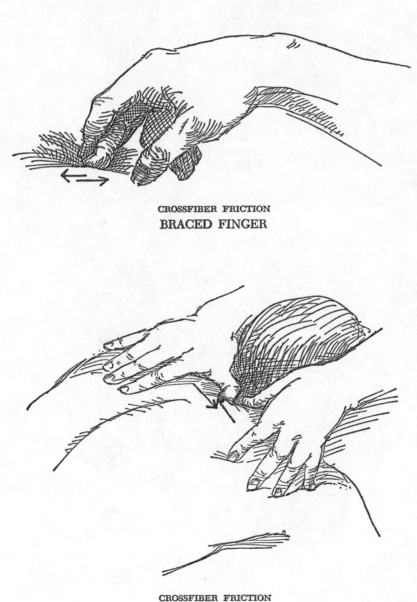

CROSSFIBER FRICTION
BRACED FINGER

CROSSFIBER FRICTION
THUMBS

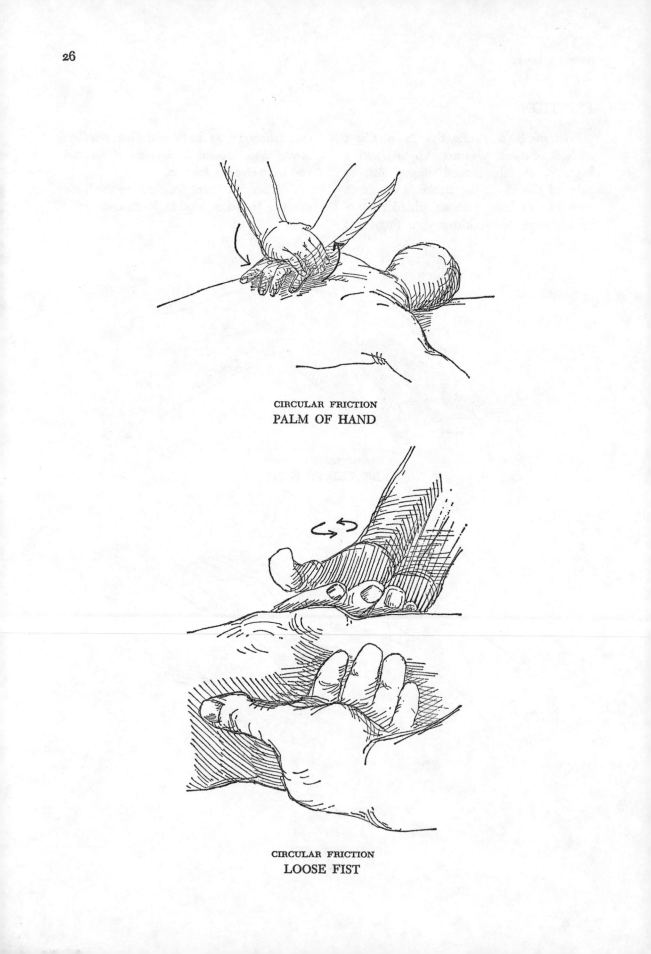

CIRCULAR FRICTION
PALM OF HAND

CIRCULAR FRICTION
LOOSE FIST

COMPRESSION

Compression movements are simply a rhythmic pumping action. The same principle of increasing depth by decreasing the area of application holds here. The muscle is compressed against its bone to achieve the spreading action. Therefore the action is always directly toward the bone.

Compressions can be applied with the fist, the palm or the heel of the hand, or with the tips of the fingers. The movement is a straight push up and down or in and out depending upon the angle of body surface you're working on.

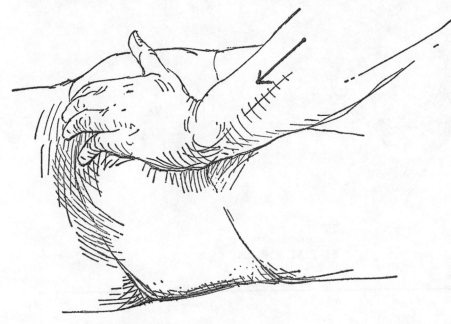

COMPRESSION
HEEL OF HAND

COMPRESSION
LOOSE FIST

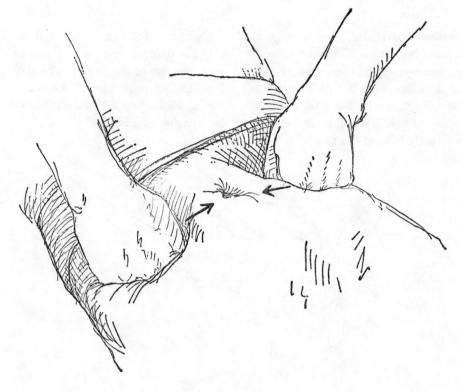

COMPRESSION
FIST AT ANGLE

PERCUSSION

Percussion is a striking movement applied rhythmically with alternate strokes. It is done with the sides of the fingers, the cupping of the palm, or with loosely clenched fists, depending on the area and the muscle mass.

I very seldom use cupping. It produces more noise than value. The important thing to remember about *percussion* is that you are not trying to beat somebody up. *This is one movement that is not directed inward.*

The full weight or impact of the hand is not allowed to follow through. The hand changes to an upward direction the instant it makes contact with the body.

Properly performed, the most rapid and vigorous movements can be applied with complete safety. To do otherwise can bruise, jar, and tighten muscles, which is the exact opposite of the purpose of massage.

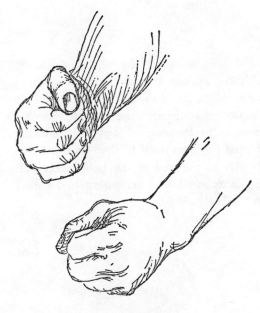

LOOSE FISTS (BEATING)

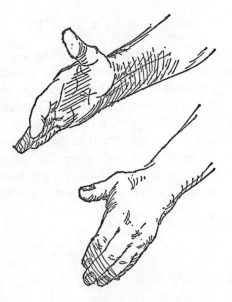

SIDES OF HAND (HACKING)

Effleurage is a sliding stroke. It feels good, it can be used to explore for tightenings, and it can spread the oil. It has its place in the treatment of fresh injuries, but it has no lasting effects and can in no way affect a healthy athletic body.

Kneading is a grasping, squeezing, and lifting motion that is relaxing to general muscle mass. However, it brings fibers closer together rather than spreading them farther apart.

In general, both *effleurage* and *kneading* may be used to relax the muscles in preparation for the four therapeutic strokes. And it is these that produce the results you want in Sportsmassage and these that should comprise at least 90 per cent of the total massage work you do.

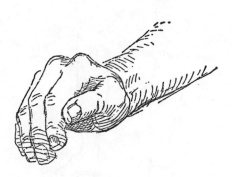

CUPPING

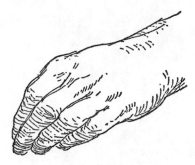

CUPPING

TOTAL BODY CHECK POINTS

The two illustrations indicate the major stress points for the entire body. It will take you two minutes or less to check yourself out for tightness and restriction before you begin to play your favorite sport.

Follow this procedure: Use *direct pressure* on each point, one after the other. Tenderness or tightness indicates potential trouble. Work on problem points in any or all of three ways: (1) By following through with the appropriate section in the Total Body Massage. (2) By referring to the chapter on your particular sport for specific therapeutic techniques. (3) By checking out the problem itself in the "On the Spot" chapter at the end of the book, where all problems are keyed according to location on the body.

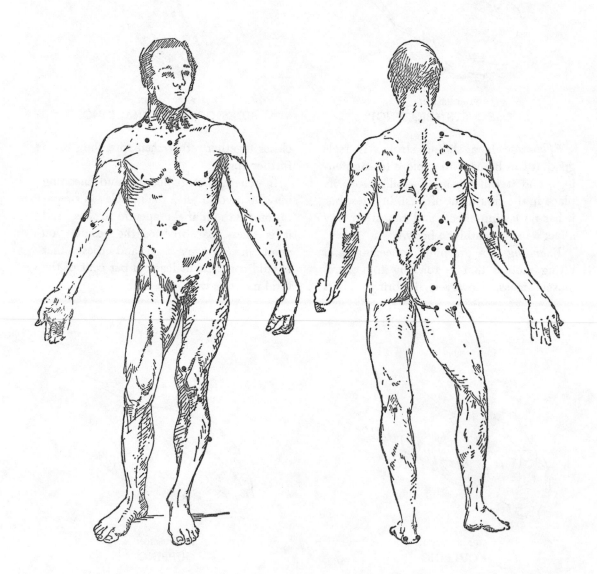

THE COMPLETE BODY MASSAGE

Setting Up the Massage

The person to be massaged should be lying face up on a massage or training table, bench, or bed. Disrobed is preferable, but by eliminating exploratory stroking, you can massage as well through light clothing. Not the feet, however: Shoes must go.

When you massage the skin directly, use a lubricant. I find peanut oil to be the best. It is a natural oil that is absorbed directly into the skin, is good for it, and leaves no greasy film. You don't even need alcohol to clean it off. Mineral oil, commonly used, is a hydrocarbon. It is not absorbed, has no nutrient value, and leaves you covered with an oil film.

THE FOOT

1. Grasp the foot firmly at the junction of the toes, keeping your fingers on the sole and your thumb on top. Make slow, deep strokes—a dozen—from the base of the toes to the heel, keeping pressure in the fingers, on the sole. The thumbs merely glide up to the instep.

2. Next, steady the top of the foot with one hand. With the knuckles of the other, press deep, stroking downward from toes to heels with six or seven passes. Apply pressure on the way down only; let go on the way up.

3. Once again, cradle the foot in one hand while you give a series of deep compressions to the sole of the foot with the other hand, using the tips of your fingers extended straight out. It takes approximately one hundred compressions to cover the entire sole.

4. Next, run your thumbs up the top of the foot to the instep, keeping in between the metatarsal bones. Grasp the foot and squeeze it firmly at its widest portion, twisting it in both directions.

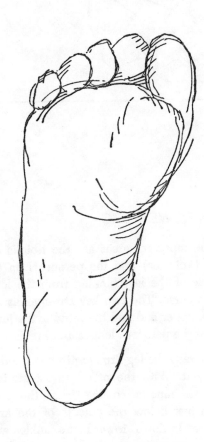

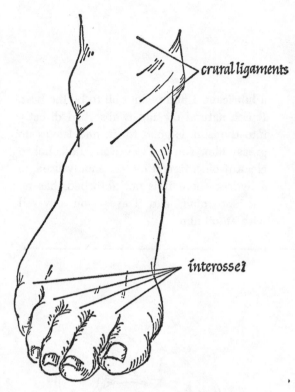

crural ligaments

interossei

5. Slide your grip to grasp all five toes and rotate them all at once—a few times in each direction. Apply a few more deep strokes as in the beginning.

6. Place the heel of the hand firmly against the instep and make deep circles to the tendons and ligaments. With the balls of your fingers make circular movements on the side areas around the ankle bone as far back as the heel. Don't slide your fingers; it hurts.

7. Last, brace the lower shin area just above the ankle with one hand. With the other, flex the foot upward, downward, and around in circles.

THE LOWER LEG

The important areas are the tibialis anticus (anterior) and the peroneals on the outside of the leg, running from the knee to the ankle. The two key stress areas are at the upper end and the middle, the junction of the peroneus longus and brevis.

1. Grasp the leg firmly with one hand to steady it. With the other, thrust straight into the muscle coming from the side. Begin just below the outside of the knee and work down toward the ankle with deep compressions applied with the heel of your hand.

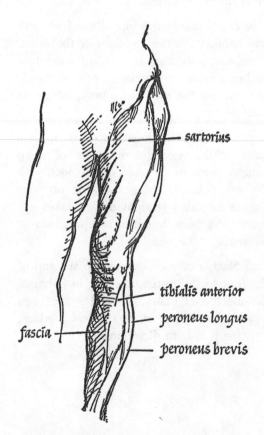

sartorius

tibialis anterior

peroneus longus

fascia

peroneus brevis

2. Ease off on the pressure about five inches above the ankle. There isn't much muscle mass there to absorb a heavy thrust. Make three passes over the entire length—twenty compressions to the pass. Increase the pressure with each pass.

3. Make three passes of circular friction with the flat of the hand to the tissue and skin of the shinbone. (For those of you who have been taught that motion is always toward the heart, this is true when stroking movements are used with venous drainage as the objective. It does not apply to compression and friction where fibers are moved in all directions.)

THE THIGH AND THE KNEE

This is a more complex structure involving the four sections of the quadriceps: the sartorius, which passes diagonally downward across the front of the thigh, the gracilis and adductors on the inner surface of the thigh-knee area, and the tensor fascia latae on the outer side. These muscles are responsible for the straightening action of the knee, drawing the leg inward and away from the midline of the body.

1. Begin by applying firm *compressions* with palms of curved hands directly down-

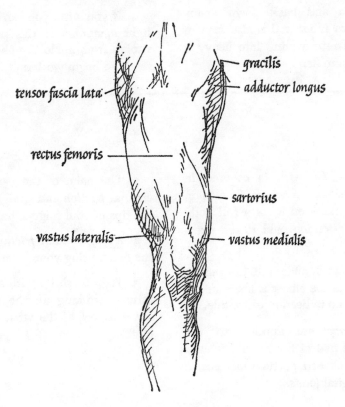

tensor fascia lata·

gracilis

adductor longus

rectus femoris

sartorius

vastus lateralis

vastus medialis

ward into the front of the thigh. Work from the top to the knee in full, generous, slow movements. This part of the body will not accept deep pressure with the heel of the hand, so modify your depth to tolerance.

Compress the area in all directions, making four or five passes down to the knee joint.

2. Then apply circular *friction* to the sides of the knee joint, first with the tips of your fingers, then with the backs of loosely clenched fists.

3. Crossfiber *friction* comes next—applied to the quadriceps expansion just above the kneecap. Work the length of your thumb back and forth across the muscle mass.

4. *Kneading* comes next—alternately grasping, squeezing, and lifting the tissue at the inner side of the knee. Work up toward the groin and back down again. Cover the entire inner and midsurface of the thigh. Moderate moving into heavy is the key to pressure here.

5. Following this, begin a series of deep *compressions*, again working up the inner thigh from knee to groin. Make three passes, twenty *compressions* each.

Repeat the same strokes on the front of the thigh, knee to hip. Then the outer side of the thigh, knee to hip. Ease off on the pressure as you reach the pelvic junction in front.

6. Once again at the outer attachment at the hip, give some extra attention—a series of deep, circular *presses* covering the entire surface.

7. The thigh is finished off with *percussion* applied first with the hands and fingers, then with loosely clenched fists.

8. Flex the knee and hip by pushing the bent knee toward the chest three times. Not rough, not fast. Just firmly and smoothly with graduated pressure each stroke.

9. If you wish, you can treat the leg to a light *effleurage* at this point—a few light strokes from ankle to pelvis. Then you are ready to begin work on the other leg.

THE ARM

Treatment for the arm is covered in depth in the section on tennis. The main difference in working on it for a full body massage is the attention paid to the stress points.

1. *Direct pressure* suffices at the points, and the tendon at the elbow is not manipulated if there is no indication of trouble.

2. *Compressions* are applied to the fingers with the pad of the thumb. Simply squeeze the thickened portions of muscle between the digital joints.

3. The palm of the hand receives both circular *friction* and straight thrusting from the tips of your fingers, held out straight.

4. Apply circular *friction* to the back of the hand, using your palm.

5. Then finish up with a series of thumb thrusts, working all the way around the lower aspect of the wrist slowly and thoroughly.

posterior deltoid

triceps

biceps brachii

brachialis
radialis

extensor carpi
radialis

extensor carpi
ulnaris

extensor digitorum
communis

extensor carpi
radialis

extensor carpi
ulnaris

THE CHEST

The important chest areas include the pectorals, serratus anterior, the intercostals, and the skin and fascia over the ribs. Stand at the side of the player's chest as you work.

1. Use the flat of one hand braced by the other to apply circular *compressions* to the pectorals, covering the upper chest from breastbone to collarbone and out to the shoulder. Take care not to touch the nipples during the massage as they are easily irritated. Work from moderate to deep pressure, keeping in mind the size and muscular development of the body before you.

2. The two key spasm areas are a point just below the collarbone about halfway between the breastbone and the shoulder and another in the belly of the pectorals approximately two inches above the nipple.

3. Move up to the head of the player and apply *compressions* using the back of your fists, loosely clenched. (No points of knuckles!) You'll see that from this position you are forcing fiber motion in a different direction than from the side.

4. Move back to the side and make large, circular movements over the rib cage with the flat of the hand. In this way you are covering both sides of the muscle.

5. Finish off with *percussion* applied with the outer edge of hands and fingers. Remember that *percussion* here should be confined to the pectorals. Do not touch the nipples. And, unless there is a specific reason for it, do not attempt to massage in between the ribs.

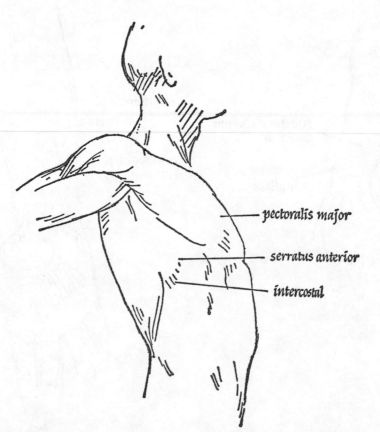

pectoralis major

serratus anterior

intercostal

THE ABDOMEN

The main area of consideration is the rectus abdominis, the main flexor of the trunk. While there are three sets of sheetlike obliques involved in the belly wall that are much concerned with twisting movements, it is the rectus that gets most of the strain. *It is also the first muscular area of the body to react to nervous pressure and tension.*

The most important part where cramping and spasm develop is the midportion covering an area from two inches below to two inches above the navel. I have come to believe this to be one of the most important points of the body, especially in the person who is tense or nervous. You will find that whenever someone has a tension headache on one side, the corresponding side of the rectus will be much more tender to pressure. When someone has been under a prolonged period of mental stress, the midportion of this muscle will be extremely painful to pressure.

Spasm here is a common cause of "false ulcers" and the gnawing discomfort associated with them. I have had customers for whom the release of spasm in this area brought an end to years of dependency upon Maalox and antacids.

Manipulation of this spot sometimes brings tears to the eyes of strong men. While working on it, I have been swung at, kicked at, and sworn at. If you let the spasm get ahead of you, the player is in for a rough time. Yet the amount of pressure you use is not that great.

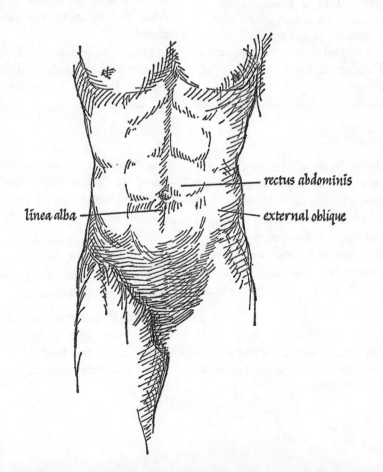

linea alba —   rectus abdominis

external oblique

I have no logical explanation for the widespread influence of this area other than the effects of nervous tension. If the rectus is not free, your body is not going to be free. It's simply true. It is interesting to me that Yoga and the Eastern martial arts all put such emphasis upon this region as a source of strength, power, and unification of the body and mind. It is your center of gravity and is influenced with every full body movement you make.

Another trouble spot here is found at the lower attachment of the rectus at the pelvis. This is strictly physical in origin and derives from stress from recovering from a backward-bend position.

1. Ask the player, still lying on his back, to bend his knees, placing his feet on the table. This relaxes the abdominals.

2. *Knead* the entire abdomen, using an alternate-hand grasping movement. *Kneading* is the most-used technique in working on the abdomen. I hope I have made it clear that *compression* requires the resistance of the skeletal structure, a requirement that immediately excludes soft areas such as the abdomen from any work of this type.

Cover the entire area, gently at first, then building up the pressure somewhat. Never be overly forceful.

CAUTION: Tenderness in the bowel can be many things. Should you come across a tenderness that seems to be non-muscular, do not attempt to work it out. Make the person aware of it and let him have it checked.

This takes care of the front half of the body. Ask the player to turn over onto his stomach now.

3. The greatest amount of *kneading* concentrates on the rectus abdominis, gripping the muscle between thumbs and fingers. Use a lifting, stretching movement and a digging-in movement. Direct downward pressure can be used from the pelvis to the navel, but never from the navel up.

4. Your finale is *direct pressure* to the stress area of the rectus by coming in to it from the sides of the muscle with the thumbs.

Five compressions, held for a period of fifteen seconds each, will cover the entire section. Pressure is to player tolerance.

BACK OF THE LEGS

Massage to the backs of the legs covers the areas from heel to hips. Because of the importance and the muscle mass, the buttocks are included in both the massage of the legs and again in the massage of the back. Mobility loss and a great many problems for the lower back and legs originate in the buttocks. It is one of the great strain areas.

1. Massage of the calf region is covered explicitly in the tennis section of the book. It is not to be ignored, and leg massage should start at that area.

2. Once you have completed the calf, move on to the upper leg. Apply *direct pressure* with the palms of the curved hands as you did to the thigh.

3. Moderate *kneading* to relieve surface kinks comes next. Work from the knee up and over the buttocks to the pelvic crest and base of the spine.

4. Starting at the lower edge of the buttocks, give deep *compressions* with the loose fist or the heel of the hand. Work down the inner aspect of the leg to the knee.

Repeat down the middle of the leg, then down the outer side. This last line is more rigid and will not accept as much pressure as the first two.

To do the job, make three passes to each line, twenty *compressions* each. Congratulations! You have worked the semimembranosus, semitendinosus, and the biceps femoris—the hamstring group.

5. Three very important points determining potential problems, or for treating existing ones, lie at the ischial origin of these three muscles. *Direct pressure* with the thumb up into the fold of the buttocks will be your method. If more than slight discomfort is felt, crossfiber *friction* should be used instead.

6. *Compressions* to the buttocks are applied with a flat-of-the-hand movement, spreading fibers in all directions. Start in the center of the gluteus maximus, the largest of the buttock muscles, and work your way up to the medius and minimum at the upper and outer quadrant.

Fifty or sixty *compressions* suffice.

7. Follow this with one more series of deeper *compressions*. Use a loosely clenched fist and cover the entire area.

8. *Direct pressure* by the thumb to the stress points is the next step. There are six such points in the area:

a. The exact center of the gluteus maximus and the underlying iriformia. When in spasm, you'll feel the pain in the lower back and have difficulty rising from a chair or low seat.

b. The gluteal fascia and lower attachment of the sacrospinalis. Again, you'll feel lower back pain and have difficulty bending forward.

c. The outer edge just above the hip joint. Spasm in the gluteus will refer pain into the lower back and down the leg. This leg pain acts much like **a**

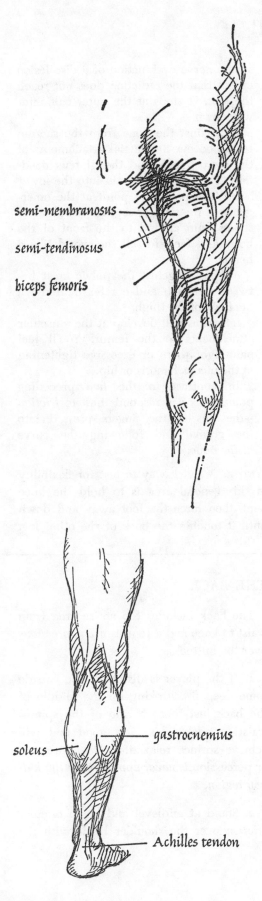

semi-membranosus

semi-tendinosus

biceps femoris

gastrocnemius

soleus

Achilles tendon

sciatic nerve dysfunction of a disc lesion except that the radiation does not reach the foot. It stops at the outer calf midway down.

d. Against the bone from the sacrum to the coccyx are fascial attachments of the sacrospinalis and the gluteus maximus. They will refer pain into the lower back. One particular point at the emergence of the sixth or seventh sacral nerve shoots pain around to the front of the body and feels for all the world like a hernia.

e. Spasm against the pelvic crest between points b and c refer pain down the front of the thigh.

f. Spasms will develop at the muscular attachments to the femur. You'll feel pain right there or excessive tightening in the biceps femoris or hip.

In contrast to the five preceding points, this one responds best to *friction* —the tips of the fingers pressed into the groove and following the curve of the bone.

NOTE: A quick way to test for flexibility in this general area is to hold the knee bent, then force the foot away and down until it touches the back of the other leg.

Then draw it up and toward you. *Gently*.

If the foot does not press down to the other leg easily, more work is required at points c, e, and f.

9. Finish off the leg with *percussion*— the knee to, and including, the buttocks. Use loosely clenched fists.

10. Bend the leg backward until the heel touches the buttocks. *This must be done with common sense*. Joint capsule "popping" has no place in responsible treatment.

Take three bends to achieve the goal. Make the first about 80 per cent of the way, the second 90 per cent, and complete with the third.

If, for those who have suffered knee damage or have had surgical repair, the resistance to bending is great, be content to stop short of absolute. You should always feel that there was a little more to be had. You can now do the other leg.

NOTE: Don't do much pressure work at the back of the knee. This is a delicate area that is better off with a minimum of work unless absolutely needed.

THE BACK

The back includes the entire area from waist to knee and a repeat of *compressions* over the buttocks.

1. If the player is disrobed, you can do some deep fist stroking up the middle of the back just to each side of the spine— waist to neck. This feels good and will achieve surface relaxation. *Deep* pressure or percussion *is never applied over the kidney region*.

2. Stand at midlevel and begin circular *friction* over the shoulder blade with the

flat of the hand reinforced by the other. Make five or six circles on each spot before sliding on to the next. Continue down the back over the rib cage.

Ease pressure below the last rib and resume it fully again as you reach the buttocks. As in all *friction* movements, the hands must not slip on the skin. The tissues must move with it. This is your preliminary loosening, and three passes down each side are enough.

3. Move up to the top of the player's head. Apply direct *compression* to the tops

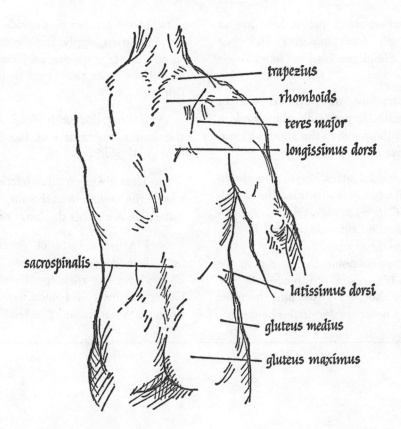

of the shoulders, for the upper trapezius and its underlying supraspinatus. *This is a most important area—one that picks up much strain and one that is always involved in nervous tension as well.*

Compressions are applied with the palm of the hand curved to conform to the contours of the body.

4. The two important points for *direct pressure* and/or crossfiber *friction* are the upper trapezius at the high point of the scapula, and the supraspinatus midway between the neck and the shoulder.

5. Give thirty to fifty deep, slow *compressions* here. It depends on the size of the player and the activity to be indulged in. Repeat the same number on the other side.

6. Then go on to give a solid thumb *press* to the stress points in the area.

7. Pick your own choice of sides and move down to rework the buttocks with a series of deep *compressions*.

8. When finished, explore the top of the pelvic crest by drawing your thumb along it from the spine out to the side of the hip. Tightenings here feel like tiny wires. These receive crossfiber *friction*.

9. Direct *compressions* with the heel of the hand begin at the waist close to the spine. Pressure here is moderate. As you move up the rib cage, you can increase it.

Three or four passes from the waist to the inferior border of the shoulder blade cover the sacrospinalis and the longissimus dorsi.

The important stress points here are at the lower rib (sacrospinalis) and just below the shoulder blade (longissimus dorsi).

10. *Compressions* now spread out to cover the entire upper back, the shoulder blade out to the point of the shoulder, and up to the base of the neck.

11. Give special attention to the rhomboids that lie below and under the shoulder blade. *Compressions* and *direct pressure* using the tips of your fingers, extended, are the strokes.

Important stress points in this region are the rhomboids, the midtrapezius in the center of the shoulder blade, and the teres major on the outer border of the blade.

12. Move around to the side once more. As you do so, apply further *compressions* to the upper trapezius and the supraspinatus. Follow the same routine on the other side.

13. Follow this with deep *kneading* to the upper trapezius and the base of the neck, both sides.

14. Then deep circular *friction* with the tips of the fingers over the shoulder blades. Take care not to hit the bony crests.

15. Finally, a taste of *percussion* with both fists covering the shoulder blades, fingers over the rib cage, barely touching. Change to heavy-fist *percussion* once more to cover the buttocks. The back is done.

THE NECK

Have the player fold his hands on the table and lean over with his forehead on them, chin slightly down toward the chest.

1. Holding the opposite side of the head for counterpressure, make *compressions* to the posterior third from the base of the neck up to the skull. You are on the upper portion of the trapezius, the rectus capitus, and the scalenus. Your pressure, while greatly modified from the back, can still be substantial.

2. Draw the thumb back and forth across these muscles, again working from the neck upward.

3. Return to *compressions*, performed with a loosely clenched fist.

Your stress points are at the scalenus at the base of the neck and on the upper attachment of the trapezius at the skull.

4. Repeat the procedure on the other side. Resist any temptation you might have to "crack the neck."

5. When the neck is completed, finish up with a series of slow, very deep *compressions* to both shoulder blades and the tops of the shoulders using the palms of the hands. I usually follow this with a shaking movement achieved by making vigorous alternating circles simultaneously to each shoulder blade.

If the person is disrobed, massage may be terminated by deep stroking from waist to neck.

The player is now expected to get up and knock the hell out of his competition!

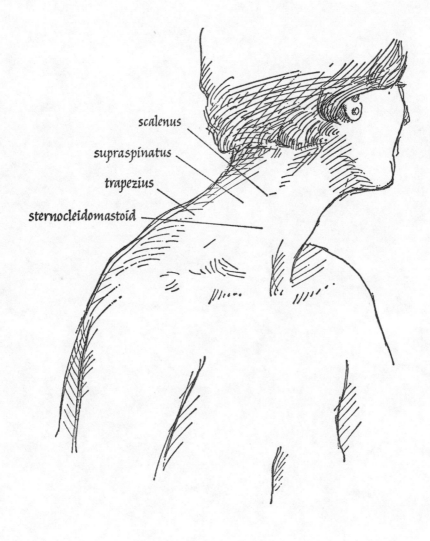

scalenus

supraspinatus

trapezius

sternocleidomastoid

NOTE: Sportsmassage can take a half hour or a full hour. There is no difference in technique between the two. While the half hour does the job, it cannot compare with the results of the hour.

There is just no way you can create the same degree of hyperemia or the durability of it in the shortened period of time.

The half hour will do nicely if the athlete is going out immediately or if the event is not overlong.

If the contest is the following day, or is exceptionally long, the hour is better. Once you have tested and felt the difference between the two, you will not settle for the shorter routine.

Part Two

Sportsmassage: The Games You Play

SPORTSMASSAGE:
THE GAMES YOU PLAY

The prime concern of Sportsmassage is to raise maximum performance levels and to prevent disablement by the increase of normal body mobility. There are many methods of preparation—exercises, stretching, warmups—all of which bring you up to your normal best.

But the deep, fiber-spreading techniques of Sportsmassage provide a synergism that gears your muscular system *above* its normal best! There is no more effective way to prepare your body for total commitment than by giving it this extra percentage of free motion.

The following sections describe how to use Sportsmassage for various sports. Very few people pay attention to prevention until they have undergone a prolonged period of physical distress. Distress has an urgency you can recognize, and relief of that distress has a tangibility you can feel.

Therefore, even though talking in terms of problems comes hard to a man who spends his life *preventing* them, the following chapters are set up to deal with major trouble spots relevant to each particular sport covered.

SOME SIMPLE SOLUTIONS

Many of the muscle problems that seem to develop for "no reason at all" are the results of a single overstretch or repeated lesser stretching of muscles not sufficiently supple. More often than not, you don't feel the symptoms immediately. You go to bed feeling fine and wake up in the morning with a stiff neck or shoulder, a pain in the lower back or somewhere else. Someone is bound to tell you that "you caught a cold in the muscle." It all seems very mysterious.

For instance, I had a client who for a period of several years, had suffered a continual tightening and discomfort on one side of his neck. It was nothing major, just a nagging discomfort. This man at fifty years of age was an excellent physical specimen and at that age was the leading scorer in a hockey league comprised of college-age men. He was a three or more times weekly customer for Sportsmassage. But in spite of the extra attention to his neck, the symptoms recurred again and again.

Knowing this man to be a strong creature of habit as well as an avaricious reader, I asked him if he always sat in the same chair evenings to do his reading. When he said he did, I suggested that he move the reading lamp to the opposite side of the chair.

In less than two weeks, the neck problem had totally disappeared. It became obvious that even the slight tilt of the head in the direction of the light had, over the period of years, caused an undue tension on the neck muscles.

Another case in point is that of a top jazz pianist who uses Sportsmassage regularly to give mobility to his forearms and hands. When he first started coming to me seventeen years ago, he was having a problem of back tightening just below the region of the shoulder blades. This was an annoying ache that would come on halfway through his night's performance. Massage would give him two or three days' respite, then the symptoms would return. My suggestion to him: Try a high seat while playing. He did and the problem left for good. What he had been doing was placing his back in an unnatural, prolonged isometric strain just holding his arms up into a position to reach the keyboard.

The Right Exercise for the Right Situation

Because what I am about to say is the opposite of accepted procedures, let me briefly reiterate the cause, physiology, and rationale of the most common muscular problems associated with sports and exercise. *The underlying cause of the muscular problem is the development of a spasm sit-* *uated at the origin—the fixed attachment—of a muscle.* The tightening and pain are transmitted to the rest of the muscle and referred to the nearest joint. The original trauma can be the result of a single overstretch, or of repeated pulls of that muscle from a lengthened position, causing irritation, inflammation, and spasm.

The accepted practice is to immediately treat the muscle injury by stretching. Stretching is fine as preparation for a contest and for prevention. Stretching is also fine after the spasm has been resolved. But during the early stages, stretching will further aggravate an existing spasm. It is, after all, what caused the problem in the first place, and to continue to stress it is the reason why many minor problems last a long time and perhaps get even worse.

What is needed during this early period is exactly the opposite of stretching. *It is contraction from a shortened angle, an activity that activates the muscle to its fullest broadening capacity without placing strain upon the damaged attachment.*

This is best accomplished by isometric contraction, using the joint limitation as the resistance. In short, exercise should be in the direction of the problem and not away from it!

It is only when symptoms have disappeared, or nearly so, that there should be a return to stretching. By understanding the kinetic principles of movement, and utilizing the stress points for both diagnosis and treatment, you will be able to determine where a problem arises. Then you can decide which is the best corrective exercise to accompany Sportsmassage treatment.

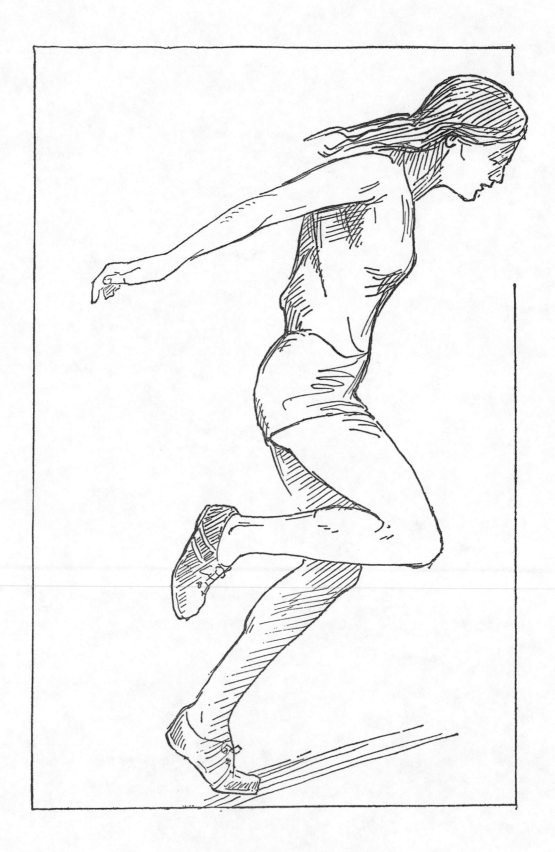

JOGGING AND RUNNING

Recently we had a blizzard here in Massachusetts that devastated the entire region. All the machinery of civilization was brought to a complete halt. And for five days only two things moved on the roads: snowmobiles and joggers!

Not many things have caught on in this country like jogging. Its practitioners come in all shapes, sizes, genders, and ages. For many, jogging has meant discovering an ability they didn't know they had: the endurance to run a respectable pace for substantial distances. New York's latest marathon drew ten thousand entrants, most of them people who entered knowing full well they had no chance of winning. But they knew they could enter and *finish*.

THE STRESSES OF RUNNING

For a jogger or a runner, the most important body area is the feet. If you do not have good feet, you will not be a good runner. In fact, if you have structurally unsound feet, you should not even attempt to be a jogger. Forget what you've heard about congenitally flat feet not causing you problems because your feet are a "natural" formation. It's bunk. The foot is the final springboard in propelling the entire body forward, and the strain on an archless foot is carried in ligaments on the inner foot and ankle.

If you find that in your running or jogging you are continuously bothered by foot, ankle, or calf discomfort, have your feet checked orthopedically. It may be a simple problem you can take care of with a fitted support—I've seen a lot of those cases. Or it may be a not-so-simple problem, in which case you'll have the satisfaction of knowing that you have averted serious damage to your most basic means of transportation.

JOGGER'S HEEL

Jogger's heel has become an increasingly frequent occurrence. Its symptoms are similar to that of a bone spur and in the absence of X ray is sometimes diagnosed as such.

Distance running, especially for those who are not good natural runners, places a great deal of repeated shock on the heel. The heel comes down solidly with each stride and this contuses and inflames the tissue at the base of the heel. This condition will be painful upon rising in the morning, will ease off after an hour or so of walking, will begin to be troublesome again as you begin to jog or run, then ease off, only to return again after you cool down.

If you press deeply into the pad of your heel with your thumb, you can feel the tightening. It feels stringy to the touch and is very painful to pressure. Usually it is found in the direct center of the heel, but on occasion you will find the sensitive spot slightly off to the left or right. Don't worry about finding it. You'll know all right when your thumb hits the spot.

Five or six minutes of deep *friction* bring immediate relief that can last up to four days. Repeat the procedure a few more times when the pain recurs until it is completely gone. Needless to say, it takes longer if you keep on running.

Jogger's Heel

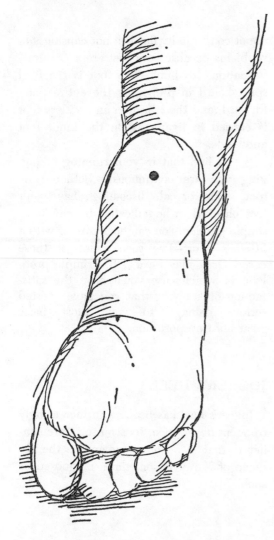

POINT 1

- Working on someone else, have him lie on his stomach with the foot straight out behind. For yourself, crossing the sore foot over the other knee is probably most comfortable.

- Use your forefinger or middle finger or thumb to probe the bottom of the heel near the center to find the trouble spot.

- Once there, apply a strong, deep *friction* to the point. Hold for a count of fifteen. Release.

- Repeat the *friction*, increasing the pressure slightly. Hold for fifteen seconds, then release.

- Repeat the two-stroke sequence again in a few days if the pain comes back, and then again if necessary, until the pain completely disappears.

CALF PULLS

Joggers do not push themselves to the extent that runners do. Therefore joggers are not commonly afflicted by the same exertion factors. Very seldom do they reach the brink of exhaustion that is an open invitation to muscle tightening and spasms.

What does crop up often enough, however, is the problem of calf pulls. This rarely happens without warning. A touch of stiffness, a little tightening when you stretch out those muscles on the downswing—these are the telltale signs announcing a muscle on the verge of spasm. You can ward off a spasm with a quick once-over before beginning to run. Take the stress points listed below and give them a couple of solid presses with your thumb. If there's pain or tightness, take a minute to two to work it out. Use the same basic routine as for an actual injury. The only difference: no pain!

The greater number of calf pulls—and the most persistent—occur on the outer side of the leg. The point to look for when you feel the cramp high up the calf is just below the outside of the knee. When the cramp is felt in the lower part of the calf, the stress point is just outside the heel. Run your fingers up and down the length of the muscle there and you find several especially tender spots and a lot of tightness overall.

Treat the problem with a combination of *direct pressure* and crossfiber *friction* on the stress points, then a working of the entire length of the muscle with *compressions*, followed by crossfiber *friction* again. Attention this time is given to the tender spots still felt throughout the length of the muscle.

EXERCISE:

From a face-down position, bend the leg at the knee to a ninety-degree angle. Flex the ankle up and down, then rotate it in a circle for a couple of minutes. This should begin "activating" the lower leg for full service once again.

Follow up with some walking, jogging, running in place, and a few toe raises. If there's no pain or tightness, go ahead and take on a mile or two of easy running.

Calf Pull

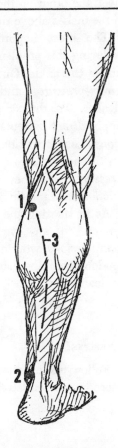

POINTS 1 AND 2

- Locate the upper stress point just outside and below the knee joint in the back of the leg. It feels stiff or tender.

- Using the tip of your thumb, apply firm *direct pressure*. Hold for a count of fifteen. Release.

- Reapply *pressure*, switching over to crossfiber *friction*, again for fifteen seconds. Release.

- Repeat the two strokes until the sensitivity of the area has decreased. It will feel easier to get into and will not be as painful. This might take several applications.

- Move down to the lower stress point at the outside of the ankle.

- Repeat the same sequence of strokes.

POINT 3

- Begin work on the entire calf muscle with a series of firm, steady *compressions*.

- Place the palm of your hand on the appropriate stress point—knee if the cramp is high, ankle if it's low.

- *Compress* the point. Count to ten. Release.

- Move your palm a bit farther along the muscle and repeat the stroke. Work all the way to the end of the calf.

- Go back to the key stress point. Place the heel of your hand on it and *compress*. Hold for ten. Release.

- Continue the *compressions*, moving the heel of the hand bit by bit along the length of the muscle. Press hard.

- Go back to the key stress point. Using thumb or forefinger, apply a deep, steady crossfiber *friction* along the length of the muscle. Hold each point for a count of ten. Then release.

- Give special attention to any tender spots you run across. An extra fifteen-second *friction* will help.

PRO TIP

In cases of severe calf cramps, it can help a great deal to insert a heel cushion in your regular street shoes. Nothing special, just the regular kind of cushion you can find in any dimestore or drugstore. Raising the heel even a fraction eases the total amount of stress placed upon the pulled muscle. Wear it for a week or so until the problem has eased up, then take it out. You want the muscle to have a chance to stretch out to its full length as soon as it can.

ACHILLES TENDON PAIN

This problem is a type of sidekick of the calf pull described above. You feel pain and a sensation of tightening in the region of the Achilles tendon just above the heel. Though the discomfort seems equally distributed over the entire region, once you find the stress points involved you have no doubt that you have reached the source of the Nile!

Like calf pull, tendonitis is one of those conditions that likes to creep up on you gradually. A little tightness at first, then finally actual hot, searing pain. It can have many causes, but the most likely is that at one time or another you came down too hard with your ankle slightly turned so that the condition is an aftershock of an earlier misstep.

When you press your fingers into the furrow between the tendon itself and the bone support to the ankle, you can feel a distinct thickness on the outer side. Probe a bit farther and you come to the two source points of the problem—both extremely tender to the touch. One is the outside of the heel, the other on the side of the leg about three inches above the ankle bone.

The most important single factor in relieving this problem is the pressure point above the ankle. On it you use a series of *direct-pressure* and crossfiber *friction* strokes. To the side of the tendon, you apply *direct pressure* and thumb *compressions*. Last, attention is given to the point on the heel, where a combination of *direct pressure*, crossfiber *friction*, and circular *friction* with the thumb is applied.

As in treating the calf pull, you should go on to an overall series of direct *compressions*, working up the length of the tendon from the base of the heel to the midcalf region.

EXERCISE:

Follow-up exercises are the same as those recommended for calf pulls.

Achilles Tendon Pain

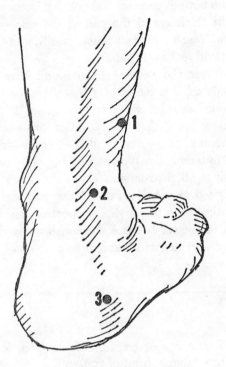

POINT 1

- Have the player stand or sit in a position where you can easily reach the tendon area. For self-massage, a crossed-leg position is easiest.

- Place your thumb or forefinger on the stress point at the side of the lower leg.

- Apply *direct pressure*. Hold for a count of fifteen. Release.

- Repeat, increasing the *pressure* somewhat, for a count of fifteen. Release.

- Apply the *pressure* one more time, pressing as firmly and as steadily as you can. Try to work deep into the muscle lesion. Count to fifteen. Release.

- Place your finger on the same spot, but use crossfiber *friction* on it. Hold it for ten seconds. Release.

- Repeat the *friction*, working deep to loosen up the stiffness beneath. Count to fifteen. Release.

- For the final pass, apply crossfiber *friction* for a count of twenty, strong and steady. Release.

POINT 2

- Find the pressure point near the center of the tendon. It will all feel stiff and swollen, but one point will be particularly tender.

- Apply *direct pressure* with the tip of the thumb. Hold for a count of fifteen. Release.

- Repeat the stroke, increasing the pressure and extending the *press* to twenty seconds. Release.

- Flatten out your thumb and apply a steady, deep *compression* to the point. Try to feel the tightened muscle fibers spreading out beneath your touch. Hold for fifteen seconds. Release.

- Repeat the *compression*. Go in as deeply as you can. Hold it for a count of fifteen. Release.

- Repeat the stroke one more time.

POINT 3

- Probe with your thumb for the stress point at the side of the heel.

- Use the tip of the thumb to apply *direct pressure* to this point. Hold for ten seconds. Release.

- Reapply *pressure*, going deeper. Hold for fifteen seconds. Release.

- Reapply *pressure*, then switch to crossfiber *friction* at the end of your press. Do that for a count of fifteen.

- Apply *friction* again. Hold for a count of fifteen. Release.

- Go on with crossfiber *friction* one more time, trying to get into the core of the muscle. Count fifteen. Release.

- Change to circular *friction*, still using the thumb or switching to your fingertip. Apply for a count of fifteen. Release.

• Finish off the sequence with one more circular *friction*. Apply to a count of twenty, working in good and deep. Release.

FOOT TROUBLES

A last foot problem common to both joggers and runners has to do with the muscles that lie between the metatarsal bones in the foot. You feel a deep cramping sensation, so deep usually that it is hard to tell whether it is coming from the top or the bottom of the foot. Both should be worked with a combination of *direct pressure* and *friction*.

On the top of the foot, you feel a tightening like a taut wire against the side of

the bone when you press into the space between the bones. It is quite sensitive. On the bottom you can feel nothing because of the thickness of the pad of the sole—until you reach the stress point, that is, and then it will feel quite painful.

Over the years I have found that the only reliable remedy for this condition is to wear a wider shoe. In the same light, I have seen that many older or heavier joggers run into trouble—literally—when they adopt the type of running shoe worn by top-flight runners. These shoes are designed to cut down on friction and weight rather than to provide support or cushion. A far better bet is a thicker, heavier shoe with greater width and more cushion at the heel.

Toe Problems

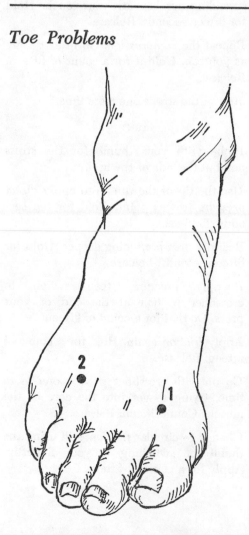

POINT 1

• Rest the foot comfortably on your knee or a table in front of you.

• Place the tip of your thumb on the stress point. It will feel tender.

• Apply strong *direct pressure*. Hold for a count of thirty. Release.

• Position your thumb on the point once again. Apply a deep *friction* up and down over the point to a count of twenty. Release.

• Repeat this two-stroke sequence five or six times.

POINT 2

• Repeat the same procedure as above.

Note that you use the same combination of strokes to handle cramps on the sole of the foot. The only difference is that you have to use more force to penetrate the thick pad of flesh beneath and behind the toes.

THE SPECIAL CASE OF RUNNING

Once you graduate from jogging to running, and especially if you begin to enter road races, you open yourself up to a much broader range of potential problems—knees, thighs, hips, and shoulders in particular. This is the point where proper warmup and prerun stretching exercises become essential.

You are also at the point where Sportsmassage delivers one of its most valuable 20 per cent extras—in the preventive, performance-boosting sense. While most of my jogging customers take their massage *after* their workout so that they can go back to work fully refreshed, most of the serious runners I deal with have learned that Sportsmassage is far more beneficial to them when done right *before* a workout or a race. They always come out with improved time and far less exhaustion than if they start out without that extra push.

Yet no matter how superbly conditioned these athletes are, things still happen. With a marathoner, for instance, the training consists mostly of fifteen to twenty slower-paced miles a day. Excepting an accident, a turned ankle, or the like, muscular problems don't develop during training as they might, say, in the case of a sprinter. The trouble generally stems from an overstretch that occurs outside of training or a difficult race that pushes the runner to the limit and causes muscle tightening or spasms.

In cases like these, checking out the major stress areas of the body with Sportsmassage is a sensible precaution. More than that if you're interested in an outstanding performance.

NOTE: For more information on the specific Sportsmassage techniques useful to the advanced runner, take a look at the following sections:

For legs, thighs, and hips, the section on soccer and the section on skating.

For shoulders and upper back, the section on weight lifting.

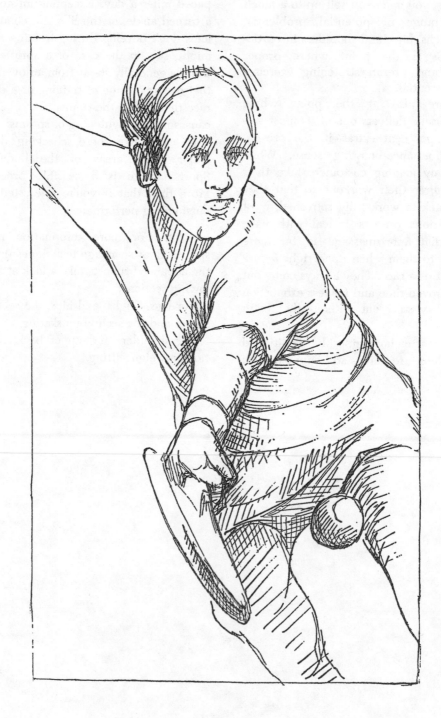

Three mornings a week I go to a tennis club for a businessman who's very much into tennis for his exercise. One day one of the pros of the club came over to me. He had been bothered for some period of time with a shoulder problem and he asked me to take a look at it for him. It took me only a few seconds to locate the trouble. He was very surprised because the muscle lesion was a good distance from where he felt the pain. Well, he knew Bob Hewitt and he told Bob about it and Bob contacted me about his own problem.

Many months earlier, he had had an elbow tendon repaired through surgery and he still could not hit a ball over one-quarter speed without intense pain in both the shoulder and the elbow. He was totally unable to return to his profession. All we had was ten days before he hoped to leave for Wimbledon and before I had to leave for the Olympics at Montreal with the U.S. equestrian team.

Now, the surgeon had done an excellent repair job on the tendon. It no longer was the cause of pain and Bob's inability to re-

turn to competitive tennis. The failure was in the postoperative therapy he had received to restore mobility to the secondary muscular lesion. That lesion had developed because of the original injury and continued to cause pain and loss of power to the arm. Muscle spasms—both in Bob's shoulder and in his arm—had started developing long before the operation. Developing while he was playing in pain from the damaged tendon.

To protect against this pain, he had altered his swing and in doing so had overused the muscles of the chest and shoulder girdle. He had lost the essential fluidity that allows maximum power to be achieved without excessive strain on an individual muscle group or joint structure.

So we began Sportsmassage treatments. By the fourth day, he was able to hit with full power and no pain. The shoulder region had cleared up completely. The arm muscles in the elbow area, weakened from disuse, required longer treatment. The heavy amount of practice Bob underwent in order to reach top playing condition caused this area to stiffen up at night. But each day the stiffening became less pronounced and we made the deadline.

While I advised him to play only the Wimbledon tournament for his safety's sake, Bob went on to play five successive ones. He and Grier Stevens won the mixed doubles at Wimbledon. On Bob's return to this country, we had another week of treatment before he and his partner went to and won the Canadian Open. When I saw him recently before Longwood, he had played forty-five consecutive tournaments around the world and was the leading rated doubles player by a very large margin.

Stress Points in Tennis

Common stress areas for the tennis player are the arms and shoulders, the calves of the legs, and the lower back. The predominant complaint in the arm is of course tennis elbow, and this chapter will deal with that problem in depth, as well as with the calf spasms that appear to be endemic to the game. Check the chapters on basketball and dancing for further development of treatment techniques for shoulder and back conditions.

TENNIS ELBOW

This condition occurs as a result of any activity that causes strain to the extensor muscles of the forearm. Strain is common in any movement that involves lifting a heavy object while your hand is in a palm-down position.

Actual elbow pain is caused by the inflammation of the tendon of origin of the forearm extensors. The elbow receives its stress from the overflexing of the wrist—as in the serve follow-through or from the repeated shock of the backhand improperly applied.

In the early stages of the condition, the combination of massage and rest can be very effective. In the acute stage, when inflammation has caused heat, swelling, and intense pain, massage may be applied to the surrounding area but not to the tendon itself. Under these conditions, massage should be used solely to restore free motion to the surrounding tissues where spasms are restricting the free interplay of muscle action.

EXERCISE:

Above all, ceasing to play before pain forces you out of the game can save you much grief and time before you can safely resume once more. What about using a forearm strap to bind the muscle? Well, it will alleviate the pain somewhat and keep you going a while longer. But this is false security. And if you incur an additional trauma to the tissue, it'll be a bad one that will cause severe damage to the tendon and will keep you out of action for a long period.

Along with the general loosening of the arm, there are five specific pressure points around the elbow itself to be massaged in order to restore free action. This is in addition to the tendon itself *when it can be treated.*

Three basic strokes are used: *compression, direct pressure,* and crossfiber *friction.* The fourth basic stroke, *percussion,* I do not use on the arm nor on any other part of the body that is under severe stress.

First, the entire arm is massaged to the shoulder with *compressions,* applied with the heel of the hand. This is to be done in two sections: the elbow to the wrist, and the shoulder to the elbow. Complete the first section in its entirety before moving on to the second.

Tennis Elbow

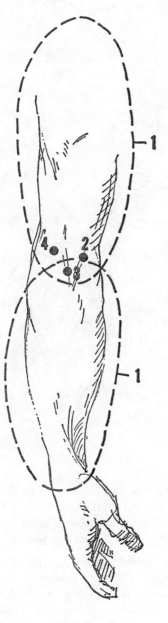

POINT 1

- Have the player place his hand palm down on a table. Fingers should be loosely spread apart.

- Using the ball of your hand, begin at the elbow to perform a series of slow, deep *compressions*. Work down the forearm to the elbow, taking about fifteen seconds to complete the pass.

- Repeat the sequence, increasing the pressure somewhat.

- Repeat it once again, with more pressure slowly and deeply applied.

- Turn the hand palm up and repeat the triple *compression* sequence. Take care to cover the entire forearm—front, back, and sides—as you work.

- Turn the hand palm down once more and begin work on the upper arm. Apply slow, deep *compressions*, working up from the elbow to the shoulder. Take about fifteen seconds to complete the pass.

- Repeat the sequence, increasing the pressure.

- Repeat the sequence, increasing the pressure. Work to feel the bone beneath the muscle mass you are massaging.

- Turn the hand palm up and repeat the procedure of *compressions*. Take care to cover all sides of the upper arm as you work.

POINT 2

- Place the hand palm up, fingers loose and relaxed.

- Using your thumb or forefinger, find the soft indentation right above the spot where the upper arm meets the inner side of the elbow.

- Apply *direct pressure* to the point. Hold for a count of fifteen. Release.

- Reapply *pressure*, working it into a deep *friction* stroke across the muscle fibers. Work for a full minute. Release.

POINT 3

- Keep the hand in a palm-up position.

• Locate the spot where the two bones of the lower arm separate about an inch below the elbow. Wiggle your thumb or finger around until you settle into it.

• Apply *direct pressure*. Hold for a count of fifteen. Release.

• Reapply *pressure*. Move into *friction*, rubbing across the muscle for a minute. Release.

POINT 4

• The hand is in a palm-up position.

• The pressure point is on the outer side of the arm where the bone connects into the elbow, again about an inch down from the joint itself.

• Apply *direct pressure* with your thumb or forefinger. Count to fifteen. Release.

• Reapply *pressure,* moving into *friction* for one minute. Release.

POINT 5

• The arm is resting on the table with the palm down.

• This pressure point is located above the elbow joint on the upper side of the bone. Find the large upper-arm bone with your thumb or forefinger. Then let your finger slip off to the side. It will come to rest in exactly the right spot, up against the bony ridge of the elbow.

• Apply *direct pressure* for a count of fifteen. Release.

• Reapply *pressure* to the point and move into a steady *friction* lasting a minute. Release.

POINT 6

• The arm is resting flat on the table in a palm-down position.

• This pressure point is the mirror image of the one above. It's just below the upper-

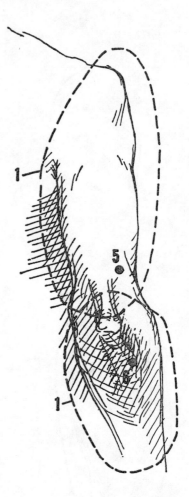

arm bone at the junction with the elbow. Press around until you find it. Your partner will let you know immediately once you find it—it's a sensitive spot.

• Apply *direct pressure* with thumb or forefinger. Count to fifteen. Release. You may notice that there's an initial sense of discomfort—not pain—when you press on this point. But it disappears as soon as a steady pressure is applied. It's a major nervous and circulatory center and as such is particularly responsive to deep massage.

• Once again apply *pressure* and change over to *friction*. Massage for one minute and release.

• Go back and run over the five stress points one more time. Apply *direct pressure* to each, but try to exert greater force than before. Hold each point fifteen seconds. Then release.

• Last, do a series of follow-up *compressions* to the entire arm. Use greater force than previously. Stretch out all your fingers and shake out all the kinks in your arm after each pass to keep your hands relaxed and responsive.

CALF SPASMS

Solid base for calf action is provided by the foot against the playing surface. The action itself is a raising of the body weight onto the surface of the ball of the foot and toes, lifting the heel up. So much of the game of tennis demands that a player be on his toes or preparing to raise onto them. It is the basic push-off position.

The greatest strain is therefore placed on the calf when it is forced into violent motion from the ready position or from the recovery from a lunge. In both instances, the knees are bent and the ankle is flexed with the foot flat on the floor.

The calf muscles are in a stretched position, with stress being placed upon the upper and outer attachments of the muscles and upon the ankle region. Injury is most likely to occur to the outside aspects of the calves because of the side-to-side motion of the body in tennis. Here the calf muscles are in constant play not only in propulsion but also in maintaining the body's balance. When strain develops, the continuous action of raising and balancing causes tightness to increase until some violent movement sends the entire muscle into spasm.

Players who bend their knees excessively in a forward-leaning posture and hold this while awaiting a serve are even more subject to calf pulls. The reason is that they are in effect holding an isometric tight contraction in the calf muscles, compounding the strain already placed on the area. Dancing in the raised-heel position also increases stress in the same region.

EXERCISE:

Lie face down on your stomach. Bend the knee at a ninety-degree angle and flex the ankle up and down, then around in a circle, slowly. Do this for a couple of minutes.

Follow-ups include some walking, jogging, running in place, and a few toe raises. If no pain or tightness is felt, go on with a mile or two of running at an easy pace if you wish.

Calf Spasms

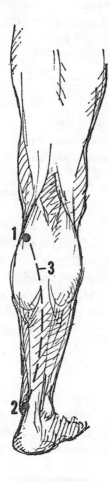

Either of these two positions provides a constant pressure that feeds an already existing spasm. The same premise mentioned earlier regarding the forearms holds true for the calves. In the well-conditioned athlete, loss of complete mobility in the hips and knees would be the factor that increases the stress in the calves and ankles; while for the poorly conditioned player, cramps develop from overuse and insufficient blood and oxygen being carried to the exercised area.

The most troublesome calf pulls occur on the outside of the leg. When you feel the spasm high up, the stress point is to be found in the lower section of the calf. When you feel it in the lower part, the stress point is just outside the heel.

The quickest way to check out the situation is to run your fingers up and down the length of the muscle mass until you find the tender, tight spots.

A combination of *direct pressure* and crossfiber *friction* is the prescribed treatment. Afterward, a working over of the entire length of the muscle with *compressions*. Then a bit of *friction* once more, concentrating on any tender spots still remaining.

POINTS 1 AND 2

- Locate the upper stress point at the outside of the knee joint. It will feel stiff and tender to the touch.

- Use the tip of your thumb to apply firm *direct pressure* to the point. Hold for a count of fifteen. Then release.

- Reapply *pressure,* switching to crossfiber *friction* as you make the point. Hold for fifteen seconds. Release.

- Repeat the same two strokes until you feel sensitivity decrease in the area. It might take several applications to reach this point.

- Move to the lower stress point and repeat the same sequence of strokes.

POINT 3

- Begin working on the entire calf muscle using a series of steady, deep *compressions.*

- Find the appropriate stress point for the problem—the knee if the cramp is high, the ankle if it's low.

- *Compress* the point. Count to ten. Release.

- Move your palm farther along the muscle and repeat the stroke. Work all the way to the end of the calf.

- Go back to the key stress point. Place the *heel* of your hand on it and *compress*. Hold to a count of ten and release.

- Continue the *compressions*, moving the heel of the hand bit by bit along the length of the muscle and pressing hard.

- Go back to the key stress point. Using your forefinger or your thumb, apply a deep crossfiber *friction* along the length of the muscle. Hold for a count of ten. Release.

- Give special attention to any especially tender spots you encounter. An extra fifteen seconds of *friction* should alleviate them a good deal.

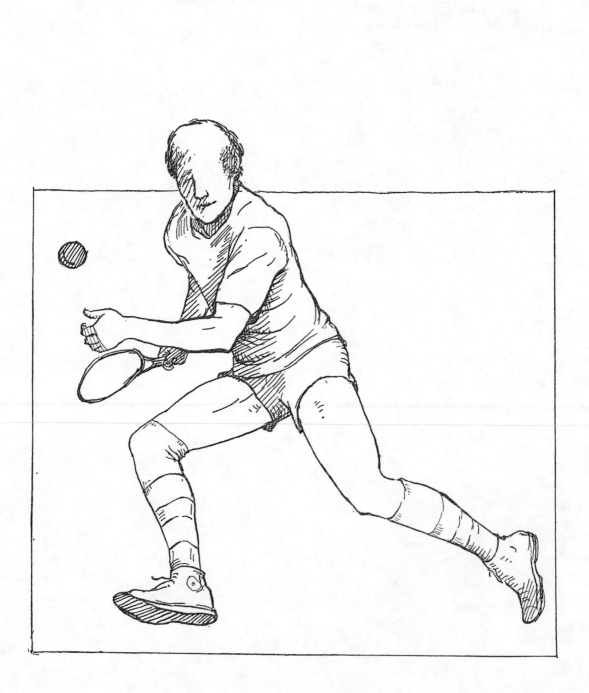

One of the fastest growing games in the country today is racquetball. It's a very fast, vigorous game that deals out a lot of punishment to the player. Already it is producing a series of specialized injuries that, curiously enough, tend to be more prevalent among the higher-level racquetball player than among those less skillful.

Though it bears an outside resemblance to tennis, racquetball is in reality a whole new ball game. In tennis, the stroke is long and flowing, a full-bodied affair that comes from a firmly planted base. The racquetball stroke is far more herky-jerky, delivered most often from an off-balance position. Its power comes from the force of the arm and shoulder region rather than as a natural extension of the entire body.

Everything is exaggerated. The ball comes from behind you and angles off all four walls. The court is small and speeds are great—in fact, the top-rated racquetball player in the country has recently been clocked at a rate of 140 miles per hour.

Areas of Stress

Movement in the sport is mostly forward and up, and backward and up. The heavy stress is felt in the arm and shoulder-support muscles. For this reason, we'll concentrate on the newly discovered "racquetball shoulder" and stress to the deltoid neck-across-shoulder area in the Sportsmassage section below. This is the section of the body you should pay particular attention to in checking yourself out before a heavy session—primarily on the back of the shoulders in an area ranging from the spine to the point of the shoulders, then down as far as three inches below the shoulder blade itself.

Additionally, racquetball demands a great deal of lunging, twisting, and bending, causing lower-back, calf, and ankle stress. We'll concentrate on twisted ankles below as well, since it is one of the most common complaints of the sport.

RACQUETBALL SHOULDER

Keith Morgan, one of my regulars, clued me in to this one. Now in his early thirties, Keith is a tremendous competitor, a real bulldog. And he's a complete racquetball enthusiast—he reads all the magazines and belongs to all the clubs.

He walked in one day with the first case of racquetball shoulder I had ever seen. Most analyses I have heard of regarding this problem concentrate on the point of the shoulder, but I have found it to be lower down, in the lower trapezius fibers. With Keith, once I took the kinks out there, the problem cleared up.

Racquetball shoulder starts as a deep ache in the shoulder blade and gets progressively worse as you continue to play. Ultimately, it becomes a constant thing that will interrupt your sleep at night and trouble you through the day even when you're not playing.

The stress point for racquetball is not a standard one included in the basic movements, but the growing popularity of the sport convinced me that it ought to be included here. You will not feel a large mass when you find the spot, but have no doubt that the reaction of the patient will let you know when you're on it!

Direct pressure and crossfiber *friction* will be used on the stress point. Then a general massage should be given to the entire back from waist to neck and out to the point of the shoulder. Use fiber-spreading *compressions* here. Finally, a checkover is recommended for the stress points of the teres major and the midtrapezius muscles on the upper midback and below the shoulder joint.

Give three or four treatments over a ten-day span. Combine this with a two-week layoff to allow the situation to cool down, then return to the game gradually. Start with a series of sessions of hitting the ball against the wall—to re-establish free movement within a safe context.

Increase the size and scope of these sessions daily until you can make the most vigorous movements *in complete comfort*. Then it is safe to return to the game. Any sooner and you run the risk of recurrence. And recurrence in this instance is worse than the original injury.

Racquetball Shoulder

POINT 1

- Have the player lie on his stomach, arms as straight out from the shoulder as is comfortable. If working on yourself, sit up straight in a backless chair.

- Find the stress point. Use your thumb or middle finger to probe the thick muscle surrounding it. Your partner will feel a sharp twinge of pain when you make contact.

- Apply *direct pressure*. Hold it for a count of fifteen. Release.

POINT 2

- Reapply *pressure* on the same spot. When you reach the bottom of your stroke, change over to a strong crossfiber *friction*. Work it for thirty seconds. Release.

- Repeat the same two strokes, increasing the pressure. Release.

POINT 3

- Begin an all-over massage of the back and shoulder region. Work up from the waist to the neck and out to the end of the shoulder.

- Use deep, fiber-spreading *compressions* applied with the ball of both hands. Work slowly, deeply, and thoroughly, covering the entire area piece by piece.

POINTS 4 AND 5

- Apply *direct pressure* to these two check points to determine any related problems.

- If pain or stiffness occurs, repeat the *direct pressure* with thumb or middle finger. Hold for fifteen seconds. Release.

- Repeat twice more, increasing the pressure each time.

DELTOID STRESS

The deltoid muscle overlaps the side of the shoulder from the collarbone down to the bulge of the biceps. It's an area that receives intense stress in racquetball, particularly as you move your arm forward from an extreme backward position. As with most other problem areas in racquetball, the major cause is the jerky speed and force necessary to play the game well.

Pain is felt in a fringe surrounding the shoulder.

The point commonly associated with deltoid strain is found at the lower end of the muscle where it attaches to the bone just behind the biceps. It is treated with a combination of *compressions*, crossfiber *friction*, and *direct pressure*.

Deltoid Stress

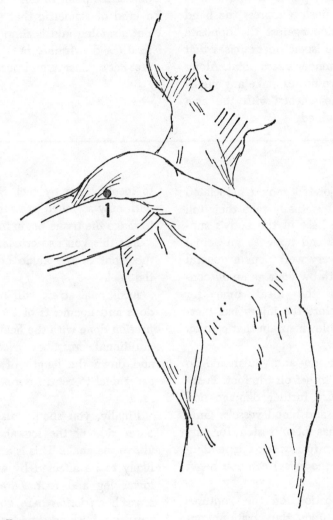

POINT 1

- Have the player sit facing a bench or table with forearms resting on it for support.

- Begin with a series of deep *compressions*. Cover the entire muscle area from the middle of the side of the upper arm to the collarbone. Use either the ball of your hand or a loosely clenched fist—whichever works better.

- Doing the *compressions* will help you to locate the spasm exactly. It will feel like a tight band running up to the point of the shoulder.

- Work up the length of the band, using your thumb to apply a good, solid crossfiber *friction*.

- Finish off with an application of *direct pressure*, firm and deep, to the stress point itself.

PRO TIP

Here are a couple of exercises to help you out with a deltoid problem:

First, a full-contraction exercise for stress point one. Press the palms of both hands flat together and push. Or press the hand of the affected side against the opposite shoulder. Both are isometric exercises that do not strain the tender stress point. Along with this, take care not to make any vigorous backward movements with the arm while it is still troubled.

The second exercise applies to the second stress point in this section. It is, again, a kind of isometric that strengthens without straining and is simply this: Stand beneath a doorframe, put your hands up to rest flat against it, and push!

TWISTED ANKLE

The rapid, disjointed moves associated with racquetball eventually take their toll at the ankles, the base of the body's support. If you don't end up with an actual sprain, you may very well incur a general stiffness that will throw your game off considerably. That's the ideal time for Sportsmassage—before the injury has blossomed into a full-blown sprain that can lay you up indefinitely.

The first thing to do—and you should do it immediately—is to get off the foot. Pushing will only cause further damage and rupture to tissues and blood vessels. Only after the ankle has been rested for any amount of time up to a week (depending on the severity of the twist) can you begin to massage it.

The actual location of the ruptures varies depending upon the position your ankle was in when you injured it. You have to locate them by feel. Start out initially with only so much pressure as is necessary to make the tissue begin to move. No more.

For this you use crossfiber *friction* from the front of the ankle bone backward to the heel.

Additional stress will occur in the tendons and ligaments of the instep. Circular *friction* done with the heel of the hand and additional crossfiber *friction* applied up and down the length of the instep do a great deal to return normal motility to the area.

Finally, you should also check out the outer side of the leg about three inches above the ankle. This is a stress point most likely to be affected by any strain on the lower leg and foot. *Direct pressure* and crossfiber *friction* here go a long way toward establishing a wider range of motion in the traumatized area.

Twisted Ankle

POINTS 1, 2, AND 3

• Have the player sit with the sore foot straight out in front, supported from beneath. For self-massage, it might be easier to cross the injured foot over the knee of the other leg.

• Use your thumb or forefinger to apply *gentle* crossfiber *friction* to the stress points just in front of and below the ankle bone, working back toward the heel. Massage each point very lightly for a count of fifteen. Release.

POINT 4

• Place the heel of your hand on the lower part of the instep. Apply gentle *friction*, moving your hand in a slow, regular circle. Work up the instep to the ankle. Sides first. Then the middle. Make each circle last for a count of ten or twelve.

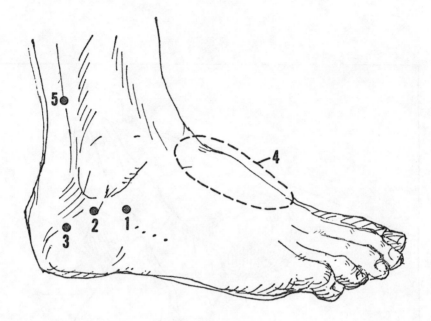

• Go back to the base of the instep. With the flat of the thumb, apply a slow and steady crossfiber *friction* at the lowest part of the instep. Don't be too rough. Work for fifteen seconds.

• Move your thumb a little farther up the instep and reapply *friction*. Count to fifteen. Release.

• Continue the crossfiber *friction*, working up the entire length of the instep on the tendons and ligaments between the long bones.

POINT 5

• Place the flat of your thumb on the stress point just above the outer ankle. Apply a steady, solid *direct pressure* for a count of ten to fifteen depending on the amount of tenderness. Release.

• Repeat the procedure twice more. Do not press any harder than is comfortable.

• Keep your thumb on the same spot and change to crossfiber *friction* for a count of ten. Release.

• Reapply the *friction* twice more, holding it for the same amount of time.

PRO TIP

One more thing: If racquetball is going to be your game, you will do well to keep yourself loose and supple. Fast movement is the most violent stress you can place on susceptible points of the body. And muscles that are going to be used fast should be trained and conditioned to accomplish such movements. I usually suggest adopting a series of karate exercises with kicks and arm thrusts swiftly performed as the best way of keeping in shape for the demands of a game like racquetball.

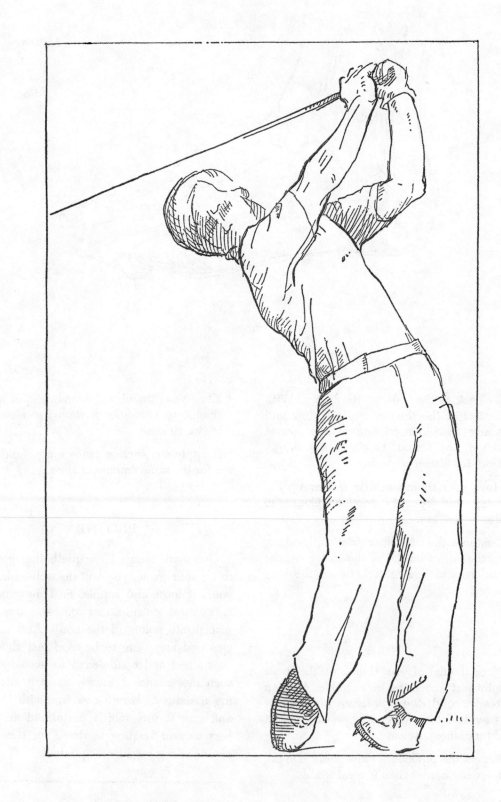

Golf is not a maximum-effort sport. It is a maximum-ability sport. Your inherent ability and how you develop it mark the sum and total of your success with the game.

Over the years I've heard golfers talk stance, grip, clubhead, arm position, whatever you can think of. All are important to the game, but each is only a part of the game. There have been only a very few golfers whom I have heard emphasize the midsection of the body as it relates to playing. And that is the key to the whole thing.

The forward slide of the hips co-ordinated with the twist of the trunk is the heart of your swing. It is also the prime area for power loss. The middle of the body transmits—and intensifies—the power generated by the legs into the region of the shoulders and arms. Anything off in timing or flexibility and power is lost throughout the entire swing.

Loss of power in this manner is such an insidious thing that you rarely realize it is happening. There is no discomfort and the body adapts very easily to the diminished situation. It always does. It seems that once a golfer accepts a certain plateau of performance, he rarely tests himself, which is a mistake. As soon as your "off days" become more and more frequent you should suspect that you have begun to lose that midsection mobility so crucial to the power of your game.

The Hackers, the Average, and the Pros

From my twenty years' association with a local country club, I have gleaned several impressions of those people who specialize in the game of golf. One is that they tend to fall into three fundamental—and fanatical—categories. There are the hackers, the average, and the pros.

I remember many years ago watching a dedicated hacker take twelve shots from the tee to the green, steering a course that would break a snake's back, and then sinking a thirty-foot putt. The twelve bad shots were completely lost in the glow of the big putt. To the hacker, all the bad shots were plain bad luck. The thirty-footer, now that was the real him!

Giving a hacker an extra degree of free motion has no value as far as improving his game. It's still lousy. No, for a hacker, the best that Sportsmassage can offer is a certain degree of comfort in which to continue to play his bad game. Bad form is his enemy, and the cause of the major part of the aches and pains suffered in the aftermath. Still, a hacker is basically a happy golfer. They play the way they want to play. And for a hacker frustration is not a byword in the locker room as it is with other categories of golfers.

Once a golfer starts to hit into the low eighties, golf stops being fun and becomes a challenge. In order to make the game more interesting, maybe you place a side bet on the outcome, and winning becomes very, very important. Losing becomes a major source of frustration, even more than an off score. Win with an eighty-nine and there is no problem. But lose with an eighty-three and the "nineteenth hole" becomes a necessity instead of an enjoyment.

The average golfer of whom we speak here has for the most part arrived as far as his capabilities will take him. Ninety per cent of the tightening problems that characteristically develop can be counted on to occur in the shoulder and neck area and lower down on the back. They are the direct result of frustration.

What Sportsmassage can do in this instance is to give you extra driving length and a longer freedom from muscle tightening and fatigue. But it can't do a thing to stop you from blowing up or missing a putt. It's a pretty vicious circle.

Logically enough, it is the professional who finds the retention of complete motion during day after day of competitive golf of greatest benefit. Look at how many times you've watched the front runner in a tournament lose it on the final day! All because the pressure finally caught up with him or her and threw off that heretofore perfect co-ordination.

Golfers, especially those in the middle group, are very fond of saying that it is a game of concentration. This is correct as far as it goes. But concentration on what? The ball? The club? The pin? No.

The top-flight golfer has all of these in the pocket. Rather it is the ability that any first-rate athlete must possess—the ability to shut off outside irritations and influences. It is not so much concentration on what is being done as *it is shutting out that which would prevent it from being done.*

As emphasized in the section on power loss earlier on in the book, when you are competing against others who have the same level of skills as you, even a slight reduction of mobility can be the difference between winning and losing. The buildup of muscle tightening can lead to a very unsatisfactory match; the retention of it, to a very unsatisfactory season.

The Sore Points of Golf

These points vary a lot, depending upon the kind of game you play. The shoulder and lower-back troubles mentioned in regard to the average type of golfer certainly are widespread. They are similar to problems that surface in other sports employing an arms-forward stretch posture. The chapters on baseball and riding cover these problems in depth.

In this section we shall concentrate on the golf-related problems associated with the basic movement most characteristic of golf—the trunk twist.

KNEE-ROTATION STRAIN

When knee strain is prevalent, the slightest amount of flexion can be extremely painful. The basic problem is that the ligaments surrounding the knee joint are frozen in spasm. Once you free them up, the relief comes quickly.

Direct pressure and crossfiber *friction* on the point of restriction are the remedies. You may have to probe around the knee joint a bit in order to find the exact point. It will be painful to the touch.

Work on the spot for a few minutes, then take a breather and test out the results of your labors. It should be very rewarding and you will see a marked increase in pain-free mobility. Try walking and a short series of deeper and deeper squats to see just how much improvement has occurred. This first session can be expanded up to three full sequences of massage, but any more than that at one time is an overdose for this kind of injury.

Lay off for a few days. If the pain recurs —and it often does in long-term cases— give it another workout. Repeat this pattern until the trouble is completely gone.

EXERCISE:

To begin, you might try a series of muscle "setting" exercises. This is a strain-free isometric that simply amounts to holding your leg with the knee straight and tightening the quadriceps (thigh muscles), holding them for a few seconds, then releasing. Ward off squat-style exercises until the condition has been cleared up for a week or two.

Knee-rotation Strain

POINT 1, 2, OR 3

- The player should sit with the sore leg stretched out as straight as is comfortable.

- Find which of the stress points is the key one. It will hurt.

- With a braced finger, apply *direct pressure* to that point. Hold it to a count of thirty. Release.

- Reapply the stroke. Hold it for the same amount of time. Release.

- Repeat the stroke once more. Hold it while you count to thirty. Release.

- Change to crossfiber *friction*. Work deep for a count of thirty. Release.

- Repeat the *friction*, increasing the pressure and the length of the stroke slightly. Release.

- Repeat the stroke again. Release.

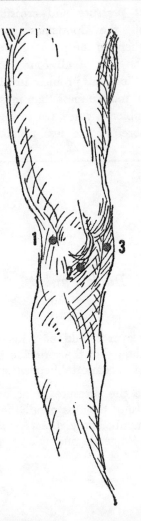

- Now repeat both the *direct pressure* and the crossfiber *friction* sequence of strokes in their entirety *twice more*.

- Stop. Do no more than three sequences at any one session.

LOWER BACK PAIN

A very common complaint is tightness and pain in the lower back region. This is a misleading complaint. The problem actually originates in the hip, where the primary stress point is located on the upper outer ridge of the hip. It feels like a cramp or a tight mass running downward toward the head of the femur, the thighbone. While you complain of lower back pain, you notice that is peculiarly one-sided. And once a bit of pressure is relieved, it becomes obvious that the trouble really lies in the hip rather than in the lower back.

Direct pressure and crossfiber *friction* lead off the Sportsmassage treatment. Apply them to the primary pressure point using the tips of all four fingers or the thumb. Since this problem involves more of the total muscle mass than most other buttock problems, you have to be more careful. Therefore use less pointed pressure, more repetitions, and less deep stroking than normal.

Move on to the strain line angling down to the head of the femur. Here you use just the opposite tack. Give it full *direct pressure* with the point of the thumb. Anything less won't have any effect on it. Then finish off by going over the same region with a series of loose first *compressions*, working it over steadily and solidly.

EXERCISE:

Trunk twisting, first from a seated and then from a standing position, drawing the knee up to the chest as though you were putting on socks, is the best way to work yourself back into a regular routine. Also walking and twisting in all directions. Avoid situps, and look around for another way to keep stomach muscles in trim.

Lower Back Pain

POINT 1

- The player should be lying on his side with the leg of the sore side brought forward in a comfortable position.

- Locate the pressure point on the outer hip. Using the tips of all four fingers or the thumb, apply *direct pressure* to the point. Be gentle but try for a steady fiber-

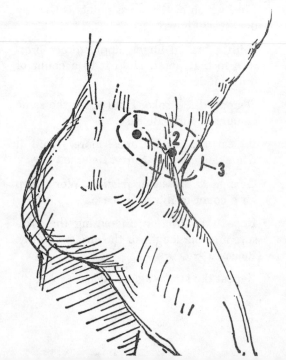

spreading press. Hold for a count of fifteen. Release.

- Repeat the stroke. Do not increase the pressure. Hold for fifteen. Release.

- Go on to repeat the same stroke five or six times. The key here is more and lighter rather than fewer and harder.

- Change over to crossfiber *friction.* Hold for a count of fifteen. Release.

- Repeat the *friction* four or five times more. Keep it steady but gentle.

POINT 2

- Locate the tight line running from the first stress point to the head of the femur. You may have to move the leg up and down a bit to get it to make itself felt, but once you've hit it you can't mistake its tautness.

- Use the tip of the thumb, positioned like a point, to work over this line. Use full *direct pressure.* Work deeply and steadily and slowly. Give each *pressure* a count of fifteen. Then release.

- Work up and down the entire length of the tight line. Then go back and give it one or two more workovers.

POINT 3

- Loosen up the entire area with a series of loose-fist *compressions.* The body surface on the hip and buttock is irregular so you have to readjust the angle of your fist as you work. Work deep and solid for about five minutes total.

PRO TIP

Here are a few words for the older golfer, those of the weekend variety, and to their club professionals. One of the most common causes of upper back and shoulder problems with this group is a direct result of a "lesson."

When your game is off, invariably the pro is going to change your swing, either flattening it out or increasing the arc. This change diverts the stress away from the portions of the muscles that have become accustomed to it and onto portions unaccustomed.

To establish this new pattern, the pro has you hit balls for half an hour to an hour using the new swing. *This is more than enough to establish a condition of overuse.* Some people will merely be stiff and sore for two or three days. Others develop spasms that do not release and invariably lead to other, more severe problems.

I recognize that the pro has his job to do and that repetition is the key to achievement. But much discomfort would be avoided by tailoring the amount of corrective work to be done to the circumstance. The herky-jerky swinger, the one with limited motion who has trouble with a backswing or follow-through, is the most likely candidate to develop this kind of spasm, and that can spoil an entire season of golf.

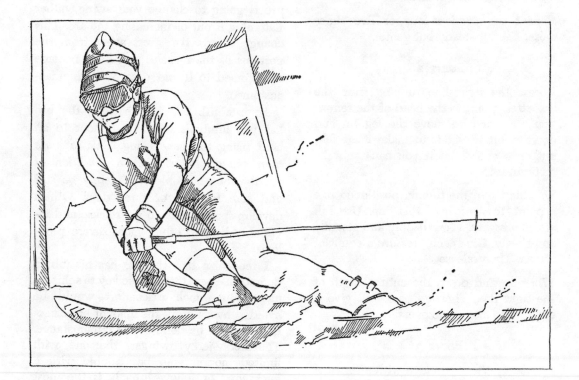

When you talk about skiing in America, you're actually talking about two very different animals. First, there's downhill skiing, a fast, demanding sport that relies on quick reflexes and perfect balance to get you down the slope in a safe, upright position.

And then there's cross-country skiing, a sleeper of a sport that's been catching on steadily over the past few years. Cross-country skiing is basically an endurance test—you against your body—where the ability to maintain locomotion for excessive periods of time is as important as technique. It is a true maximum-effort sport that falls into the same category as marathon or cross-country running. And, as in these sports, the leading villain is the same. It is the muscle-tightening barrier that the skier must break through or push back if he wants to successfully complete his course.

Cross-country involves no overstretches. Rather, the aching and tightness that develop in your shoulders, lower back, stomach, and legs are the direct result of our old friend glycolysis—meaning too little oxygen and too much lactic acid.

At first, the spasms are minimal and your absorption with the terrain and the business of skiing are sufficient to make you overlook them. But each time you ski, those spasms will feed upon themselves and enlarge, taking up more and more of power supply until you think you're simply in a slump, tightening sooner and tiring quicker.

Downhill Skiing

Downhill skiing demands lightning reflexes for instantaneous changes of direction, coping with unforeseen obstacles, and traveling at a high rate of speed. The weight shift demands compensatory action from the entire muscular system. The raising of an arm or a forward bend from the waist each require multiple simultaneous contractions in widely ranging muscle groups in order to provide a counterbalance.

Thus, while the downhill event is not of long duration, the body is in constant isometric contraction while it is being performed. This type of contraction inhibits circulation and produces a serious strain on the muscles involved.

As the tightening process gains momentum, reflexes, co-ordination, and balance deteriorate. And it explains the skier's fact of life that more broken bones occur during that "one last time" down the slopes than at any other time.

Areas of Greatest Stress

The neck and shoulder region, in skiing, come in for a heavy dose of overstrain due to the locked posture in the bent-forward position. The tension you experience is very much like that of a horseback rider. The chapter contains a thorough description on Sportsmassage techniques designed to deal with this particular condition.

Below the shoulders, it is the hips, lower back, and thighs that are most heavily stressed in skiing. Since strain to these areas comes on so insidiously, it is even more crucial than normal that you maintain a close check on the stress points affected each and every time you go out to ski.

THIGH SPASMS

A compound problem involving the knee joint and the quadricep muscles in the thighs produces this familiar skier's complaint. Pain is felt in a pull around the knee when walking down stairs or down a hill, and there is a general tightening at the top of the knee joint that, when investigated, spreads all the way up the front of the thigh.

Treatment consists of *direct pressure* and crossfiber *friction* applied at six stress points circling the knee at a radius about 1½ inches beyond the joint. Continue with crossfiber *friction* down the sides of the knee joint to relieve any stress to the various points of attachment there.

Last, go over the entire surface of the knee with a round of circular *friction,* using first your fingertips and then the loose fist.

EXERCISE:

Muscle setting—tightening the quadriceps with the knee held straight—is the proper exercise in this initial period. Don't try any repetitive squats until the condition has cleared up completely.

CAUTION: In any instance where it is painful to straighten the leg—or if you can't straighten it at all—you have to consider the possibility of deeper trouble, such as cartilage damage. Have it checked out by an orthopedist. The knee is a much more complicated joint than it appears to be, and any injury involving more than simple strain should receive prompt medical attention.

Thigh Spasm

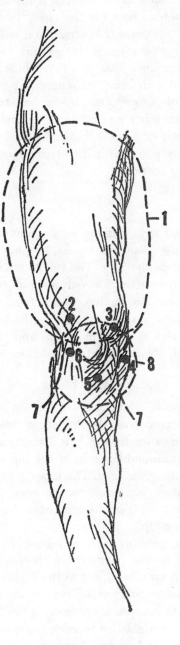

POINT 1

- Have the player lie face up with the leg out straight.

- Begin by freeing up the entire thigh area with a general Sportsmassage, as described in the chapter "How to Do It."

POINTS 2 TO 6

- Locate these points, one by one, with the point of the thumb or a braced finger. They will be sore when you hit them.

- Apply *direct pressure*, holding for a count of twenty. Release.

- Repeat the stroke, increasing to twenty-five seconds.

- Repeat once again for a count of thirty. Release.

- Change to crossfiber *friction*. Work for a count of twenty. Release.

- Repeat the stroke, increasing it to a count of twenty-five. Release.

- Repeat once more. Hold to thirty. Release.

- After the first sequence, test out the leg for improvement. Is it less sensitive to pressure? Can the player do a full, painless squat? If the answer is yes, quit.

- If no, repeat the *pressure-friction* sequence two more times, maximum, and let it go for the day. Don't overwork the knee—ever. Try it again the next day.

POINT 7

- Apply a slow, steady crossfiber *friction* down both sides of the knee joint, working out any additional trauma built up here.

- Repeat the pass if any area is especially tender. But take care not to apply any more pressure than is comfortable.

POINT 8

- Finish off with some attention to the total kneecap area. Apply a slow, solid, circular *friction*. Use first your fingertips, then a loose fist. The surface is bony and irregular here, so have your hand nice and relaxed to accommodate the contour of the knee.

LOWER BACK AND HIP PAIN

A sport with as much trunk twisting and bending as skiing puts a lot of wear and tear on the muscles of the lower back and hip. Consequently, a lot of stress points are involved here, and in order to determine exactly which ones pertain to your particular problem, you have to test them all out. Think of it like going to one of those test-it-yourself gizmos for radio tubes they used to have in the drugstores. Press the tube in and if it doesn't light up, it's dead, or, in this case, press on the point and if you don't light up—with pain—it's okay.

Anyway, the sequences described below cover all of the trouble spots in the lower back-hip region. It won't hurt to Sportsmassage the entire sequence, but you can pick and choose the ones that need it the most at any given moment.

Stress Area One

The first major stress point is the one on the extreme outside of the hip. When this one is "on," you feel tightening and discomfort down the leg as well as in the lower back, particularly on the one side. A general Sportsmassage loosening of the entire buttock is in order, followed by *direct pressure* and crossfiber *friction* on the point itself, angled from the side for better contact.

Pain down the leg indicates bigger trouble, so a series of *direct presses* with the thumb all down the outside of the leg is performed. Along the way you will find two tender spots—one at the outside of the knee and the other at midcalf. Give an extra minute of *direct pressure* here. While doing this, return to the original stress point five or six times and give it an extra bit of *direct pressure*. Pain of pressure will be dramatically reduced after the second or third trip back.

Stress Area Two

Dead center in the buttock is the second major trouble spot for the lower back-hip area. If this point is in stress, you will feel it when you attempt to get up from a seated position. This is a superthick area, particularly in heavy or muscular persons, and requires more pressure for penetration than most other areas. So use the point of the thumb or braced fingers to work over the stress point with *direct pressure* and crossfiber *friction*.

EXERCISE:

Start off with walking, sitting, and rising from a chair, and full squats, keeping your heels flat on the floor. The squats are not a repetitive exercise. Do only enough to establish painless motion. Aside from that, just normal walking—increasing the length of the stride—and going up and down stairs will give sufficient, strainless exercise.

Stress Area Three

This point, on the side of the hip about one inch away from the first one mentioned here, comes on feeling like a tight cramp that runs around the side of the hip down toward the groin area. The lower back can hurt, but as you work on the area, you'll find that it really is radiating from that one side of the hip.

Direct pressure and crossfiber *friction* are used on the point, but with less pressure than on other spots in the region due to the wider amount of muscle mass involved. An exception, however, is the treatment of the tight line running down to the head of the thighbone. This you treat with full *pressure;* it's usually that hard.

EXERCISE:

The best exercise for this area is twisting your trunk from a seated position. Then twisting your trunk from a standing position, drawing your knee up toward your chest as if you were putting on a sock. By

all means, avoid situps. They are disastrous for a lower back condition of this nature.

Lower Back and Hip Pain

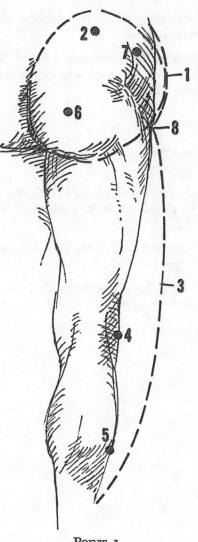

POINT 1

- Have the player lie face down, legs out in back as comfortably as possible. If tense in the buttock region, have him cross his sore leg over the other one at the ankle. It helps.

- Work over the entire buttock region with a general massage, as described in the chapter "How to Do It."

POINT 2

- Apply *direct pressure,* using the point of the thumb to the point. Coming at it from the side gives you surer contact. Hold for a count of fifteen. Release.

- Repeat the stroke. Increase to a count of twenty. Release.

- Repeat the stroke, inceasing your hold to twenty-five. Release.

- Switch strokes to a crossfiber *friction.* Hold for a count of fifteen. Release.

- Repeat the stroke, increasing the hold to twenty. Release.

- Repeat the stroke again. This time hold it for a count of twenty-five. Release.

- Return to this stress point with additional *direct pressure* five or six times more during the course of the next several strokes. You will find the sensitivity greatly reduced with each succeeding pass.

POINT 3

- Go on to apply *direct* thumb *pressure* down the outside of the leg. Hold each point for a count of ten before releasing and moving on to the next. Two tender spots will be found.

POINT 4

- The first of these tender spots is on the outside of the knee. Apply further *direct pressure* here. Work for a minute, taking a rest between presses.

POINT 5

- Treat the second sensitive spot in the same manner—*direct pressure* off and on for a minute—applied to the point at the outside of the middle of the calf.

POINT 6

- Locate the pressure point in the middle of the buttock. It feels like a tight ball or a mass of strings.

- Apply a deep *direct pressure*. Hold for a count of fifteen. Release.

- Repeat the stroke. Increase the hold to twenty. Release.

- Switch to the crossfiber *friction* on the same point. Hold for a count of fifteen. Release.

- Repeat the stroke, increasing the time of the hold to twenty. Release.

- Go back to this point with further *direct pressure* several times more during the rest of the massage. Keep trying to go deeper. It will feel better each time.

POINT 7

- Apply *direct pressure* to this point with the thumb or tips of the four fingers. Hold for a count of fifteen. Release.

- Repeat the stroke, increasing the hold time to twenty. Release.

- Go on to crossfiber *friction*. Hold this for a count of fifteen. Release.

- Repeat the *friction*. Increase the hold to twenty. Release.

- Return to this point again before finishing up. More passes, less depth are the keynotes here.

POINT 8

- Locate the tight line running down from the previous point.

- Apply full *direct pressure* with the point of the thumb. Hold for a count of fifteen. Release.

- Increase the time of the stroke to twenty and repeat it.

- Continue the deep *pressure* all the way down the length of the spasm.

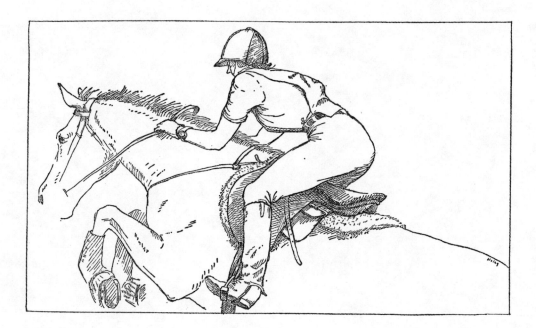

The uninitiated have a tendency to regard horseback riding as a nonstrenuous activity where the horse does all the work. Not true. Of course, much depends upon the type and the degree of riding you do in the same way that much depends upon the type and degree of any sport you participate in. And for sure the greatest danger in walking out a tired old nag is that you'll fall asleep and tumble off. A spirited horse is something else again!

In my capacity as sportsmasseur for the United States Equestrian Cross-Country Team and with my work with race horses, I see continual evidence of the strain factors that occur to riders both off and on horses. To begin with, I've worked on stress points on the team horses as sore as any human athlete's can get and have felt under my own hands the response you get when push comes to shove with fourteen hundred pounds of horseflesh behind it. The experience has left me with a healthy respect for the men and women whose business—or passion—it is to work with these giants on a regular basis.

The Rough Points of Riding

Controlling three quarters of a ton on the hoof at a gallop, over a jump, or across rough terrain is as physically demanding as any sport can be. It uses the entire body to do it well. And it causes intense pressure in several specified areas of the body.

The control factor alone—pulling on the reins—for any length of time severely aggravates the region across the back of the shoulders. Farther down, the lower back comes in for its share due to prolonged forward bending.

The ultimate *coup de grâce* for a rider, of course, the one injury that no amount of tape or no number of pain pills can ultimately subdue, is the severe groin pull. Common enough to have been chronicled as "rider's muscle," groin pull is a result of abuse suffered over hours of isometric tension in a riding posture.

Another major contributor to stress problems in riding is the inordinate number of broken bones and torn ligaments that accrue to those who jump, hunt, and otherwise go cross-country with horses over rough terrain. The adhesions and secondary lesions surrounding old injuries make the entire area far more susceptible to tightening and stress. Increasing the mobility of these areas with Sportsmassage lessens their potential for subsequent reinjury in a new stress situation.

PRO TIP

This is not so much a pro tip as a pro tidbit of interesting information. I ran across a very interesting study a few years ago comparing the cardiovascular systems of various types of athletes. Well, with all the current emphasis on running for your life, I felt sure that runners, especially long-distance runners, would come in easily with top honors. The surprise was that jockeys were the winners by a wide margin. Naturally, the size and the necessity for maintaining minimum weight are factors here. But the amount and variety of physical activity associated with horses (most riders, you know, care for and clean up after their own horses) are integral parts of the sport.

BACK-OF-SHOULDER STRESS

The two most common stress points in the shoulders are found at the top of the shoulder blade and, farther down a couple of inches, right in the middle of its edge. Spasm in the upper point (the upper trapezius) is felt in the neck and head. If you're a person susceptible to headaches, it'll probably crop up there, giving you pain up the same side of the head as the shoulder is on and possibly clogging that nostril as well.

It's likely you'll have a stiff neck as well. And the treatment here is crossfiber *friction* applied to both the stress point and the junction of the neck and shoulder.

The point in the center of the shoulder blade, the midtrapezius, receives the brunt of the stress in riding due to the isometric contraction you hold the muscle in as the horse pushes against the reins. The lesion that develops here is one of the most painful ones to work on, and when it is under severe stress, the pain will be referred all the way into the arm. Even after you're off the horse, you still feel a tingling or numbness in the hand.

Tandem to strain in the midtrapezius is strain in the teres muscle, at the back where the arm connects to the torso near the armpit. It is most likely to be the culprit when the pain is felt in the upper arm, between the shoulder and the elbow, whereas the first point is responsible for pain or tingling all the way down in the hand.

CAUTION: When symptoms reach down into the hand, it is very important to have a logical reason why. If you have had a fall, a blow to the head or to the neck, or have a history of neck problems, go to an orthopedist or neurologist posthaste! The symptoms are similar to those of a cervical disc lesion. Don't take chances. Rule out the more serious possibility first.

The lesion feels like a tight line running from the middle of the shoulder blade out toward the shoulder. One spot in particular will be very painful, and that is where you go in with *direct pressure* and crossfiber *friction* first. It hurts like hell and there is no way around it except to break off every once in a while. I've been called some pretty choice names while working on this one and only the fact that results come quickly has prevented mayhem by some of my larger and tougher customers!

The entire shoulder blade is treated by *compressions*, but you have to keep returning to the hurtful point as well. While relief can be obtained very quickly with the *direct pressure*, you need at least fifteen or twenty minutes to produce long-lasting results.

The point on the teres can be reached from the side. The muscle here is full and requires more pressure than the former area worked on. *Direct pressure* is best applied with the point of the thumb; and crossfiber *friction*, by a to-and-fro movement with the thumb hooked over the outer edge of the shoulder blade.

EXERCISE:

The follow-up exercise is simply pressing the arms backward and downward. No forward or upward stretching is done at this time.

Back-of-shoulder Stress

POINT 1

• Have the player lie face down with the hands underneath the forehead.

• Apply crossfiber *friction* with the tip of the thumb or braced forefinger. Hold for a count of fifteen. Release.

• Repeat the stroke for a count of twenty. Release.

• Repeat the stroke one more time, holding for a count of twenty-five. Release.

POINT 2

• If a stiff neck is a symptom, go on to apply crossfiber *friction* to the junction where the neck and shoulder meet.

• Use your thumb flat, or the fingertip held in the same position. Hold for a count of fifteen. Release. Work in a circle, covering the entire area.

POINTS 3 TO 4

• Locate the painful center stress point.

• Apply *direct pressure* for a count of fifteen. Release. Relax between strokes, remembering that this is an especially painful area.

• Repeat the stroke, increasing to twenty. Release. Wait a minute.

• Repeat the stroke again. Count to twenty. Release.

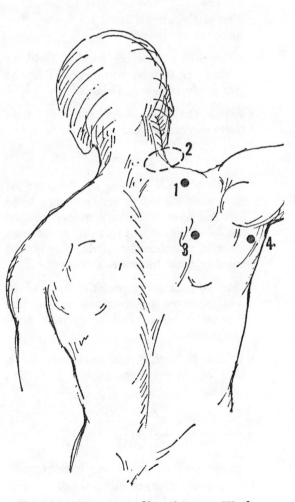

• Change over to crossfiber *friction*. Work to a count of fifteen. Release. Wait.

• Repeat the stroke, increasing the time to twenty. Release. Wait.

• Repeat the stroke again. Count to twenty. Release.

POINT 4

- Locate the teres point on the underrim of the shoulder blade. Approaching from a side position is easiest.

- Apply *direct pressure* using the tip of the thumb to penetrate the heavy muscle tissue here. Hold for a count of fifteen. Release.

- Repeat the stroke, increasing the count to twenty. Release.

- Repeat the stroke. Hold for twenty-five. Release.

- Change to a crossfiber *friction*. Hold for a count of twenty, working as deep as you comfortably can. Release.

- Repeat the stroke twice, extending it to thirty seconds. Release.

POINT 5

- Finish off with a series of *compressions* done with the flat of the hand or a loose fist. You have to be very relaxed so that the hand conforms to the irregular contours of the shoulder blade. Slowly and steadily, cover the entire shoulder blade.

- Now go back and repeat the series of *direct pressures* and *frictions* on the first four stress points. Follow up with more *compressions*.

- Follow through these sequences for a total of twenty minutes the first time around.

LOWER BACK PAIN

In the midback and lower back regions, the isometric strain of riding is felt first just below the shoulder blade where the latissimus dorsi has its upper origins. You feel the discomfort right there. Sometimes it reaches all the way around to the front of the chest where it spasms each time a breath is drawn.

Sportsmassage concentrates first on the stress point itself, applying a combination of *direct pressure* and crossfiber *friction*. From there you work down the length of the muscle, first with *compressions,* then more pointedly with crossfiber *friction*.

About halfway down the muscle you find a strip of four inches or so in length that is supertender. Treat that section with further crossfiber *frictions*. *Frictions* again are prescribed for working out any additional lesions in the nearby muscles (the rhomboids) lying just under the edge of the shoulder blade.

Lower Back Pain

Lying just below the last rib is the key stress point for pain in the lower back region. A couple of inches below is located another major point—one of the trickier ones to handle. It lies just below the bony ridge of the pelvis, and the reason you have to be careful here is that when you first run across it, in spasm, it feels stiff and hard. This is deceptive, because it is actually a very vulnerable area with no bony or heavy muscle protection of its own. The kidneys lie directly between the two points where much of the generalized spasm occurs. *Never handle it roughly, and under no circumstances ever use* percussion *in this region.*

To the two stress points, you apply the standard effective combination of *direct pressure* and crossfiber *friction*. Then work over the entire buttock region with *compressions.*

The first time through, the three-stroke sequence is done with minimal pressure. You repeat it several times over, if necessary, increasing the pressure *only to tolerance.* It will improve measurably, but during the first session will never completely clear up. Leave it after several passes, and come back to it at a later date.

Lower Back Pain

POINT 1

- Have the player lie on his stomach, the arms under the forehead.

- Find the stress point, a small nodule about 1½ inches below the lower, inner corner of the shoulder blade.

- Apply *direct pressure* with the thumb. Count to fifteen. Release.

- Repeat the stroke, holding for a count of twenty. Release.

- Repeat the stroke. Increase the time held to thirty seconds. Release.

- Apply more *direct pressure,* in the same time and pressure sequence as with the preceding stroke. Release.

- Change to crossfiber *friction.* Use your thumb or a braced forefinger. Hold for fifteen seconds. Release.

- Repeat the same stroke. Hold for a count of thirty. Release.

POINT 2

- Use the flat of your hand to perform a series of *compressions* down the length of the muscle.

- Change to the heel of the hand. Repeat the *compression* sequence. Work slowly and deeply.

- Do one more pass with the heel of the hand. Work in as solidly as possible.

- Use your thumb to apply a deep crossfiber *friction* along the outer edge of the muscle. Take your time and work as deeply as you can.

POINT 3

- Find the sensitive stretch of the muscle— an area about four inches in length somewhere near the middle of the muscle.

- With the thumb, apply additional

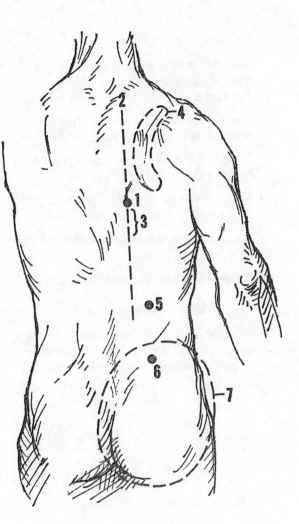

crossfiber *frictions* here. Count to fifteen for each stroke. Then release.

- Repeat the sequence one more time.

POINT 4

- Press your fingertips or thumbs deep into the furrow behind the shoulder blade.

- Apply a solid crossfiber *friction* all along here. Work slowly and deeply. Count to fifteen. Release.

- Repeat the stroke, increasing to a count of twenty-five. Release.

POINTS 5 AND 6

- Use your thumb or forefinger to apply *direct pressure* to both of these points. Hold for a count of fifteen. Then release.

- Reapply the stroke, increasing the time to twenty-five seconds. Release.

- Repeat the stroke once more. Hold to a count of thirty. Release.

- Switch over to crossfiber *friction*. Hold for a count of twenty. Release.

- Repeat the stroke for a count of thirty. Release.

- Repeat the same stroke once more.

POINT 7

- Using the palm of your hand, begin a slow, steady series of *compressions*. Cover the entire area of the buttock.

- Repeat the series, this time using the heel of the hand.

- Finish up with one more round of *compressions*, this time using loosely clenched fists.

GROIN PULL

Groin pull can be a total nightmare for the competing rider. It's a fact of the game that when you ride a horse, you grasp it with your legs. It is bad enough merely spreading your legs apart with a groin pull. To jump or to gallop a horse—where you have to squeeze—is excruciating.

Treating groin pull is a painstaking process. The full treatment for this problem can be found in the chapter dealing with soccer.

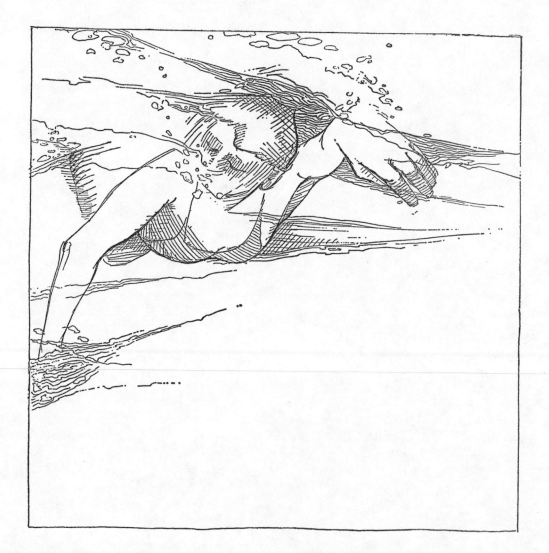

Swimming is a maximum-effort sport. Like running, it's the low-oxygen/lactic-acid buildup that breaks you down, rather than actual injuries.

The pain of maximum effort can be greatly eased by a few passes of Sportsmassage before an event. The pain comes from your body fighting its built-up resistance. Reduce that resistance and not only do you relieve the pain, you also improve the time.

Trouble Spots

I have met former swimmers who have told me that for years after they had ceased to swim, they were still subject to discomfort around the shoulder blades, and that this trouble would reappear at the slightest provocation, just as surely as it had plagued them all the while they were active in the sport. And they wondered why.

The reason, of course, is that the old lesions have never been worked out. And certainly the area of greatest concern for swimmers is the trapezius of the upper back and shoulder. Add the lower back for specialists in butterfly.

The hamstrings should also receive special attentions for all swimmers, not so much that they will cramp during the event, but that they will cause trouble in later years. Swimming is a sport with unusually long-lasting results. Your body remembers its swimming injuries long after you have packed their memories away with your old tank suit.

The reason why is that in swimming the legs never receive any degree of forward movement. Therefore the successive tightening develops shortening of the muscles, which makes them more susceptible to injuries from outside movements, especially in later years. One way to avert the problem is to give close attention to the hamstring muscles of the thigh. The chapter on basketball contains a full description of check points and Sportsmassage for hamstrings that would be of use to the swimmer as well.

PRO TIP

A word on exercise—stretching exercise in particular—and swimmers. Sprint swimmers are less liable to run into the kind of hamstring and long-run leg trouble described above. For one thing, they tend to be more lean and flexible due to the rapid movements required by their specialty. Also, their training routine regularly includes stretching.

Distance swimmers, on the other hand, are more heavily muscled. Their stroke is much slower-paced, and endurance rather than speed is the key factor. Notoriously, as well, they are much less likely to include adequate stretching movements. If distance swimming is your thing, now, while you are doing it, is the time to compensate for future leg trouble. Include stretching in your regular workout and take up the appropriate Sportsmassage routines to ward off foreshortened muscles.

SHOULDER TROUBLE

Swimmers can look for the seat of their shoulder problems at two stress points: one at the top of the shoulder blade, the other a couple of inches farther down, in the middle of the edge of the blade. Trouble in the upper point is referred to the head and neck in the form of pain and stiffness.

Prescribed treatment is crossfiber *friction* right on the point and also at the part of the shoulder where it meets the neck.

The point in the center of the shoulder blade, the midtrapezius, is a major source of spasm in swimmers. It is also one of the most painful spots on the body when in spasm. The pain here shoots down into the arm, sometimes causing a tingling sensation in the hand itself.

A third related stress point is found on the back just under the arm. This is the teres muscle, and spasm here is felt primarily in the upper arm—between the shoulder and the elbow. Between the teres and the trapezius runs a tight line. It is very painful, and even the tenderest *direct pressure* and crossfiber *friction* draw complaints. The only way to handle it is to work a little, lay off a little, then work a little more.

The stress point teres itself gets *direct pressure* applied with the point of the thumb from the side. Follow up with crossfiber *friction*, using a back-and-forth movement with the thumb hooked over the outer edge of the shoulder blade.

The final stroke is an all-over massage of the entire shoulder blade using *compressions*. After that, you can repeat some of the earlier strokes for additional relief.

EXERCISE:

Very simply, all you can, and should, do at this point in the way of exercise is to press your arms backward, then downward. Do no forward or upward stretching at this time.

Shoulder Trouble

POINT 1

- Have the player lie face down, hands beneath the forehead.

- Apply crossfiber *friction* with the tip of the thumb or braced finger. Hold for a count of fifteen. Release.

- Repeat. Hold for a count of twenty. Release.

- Repeat. Hold for a count of twenty-five. Release.

POINT 2

- Where a stiff neck is a problem, go on to work on the junction of the neck and shoulder with crossfiber *friction*.

- Use the thumb flat, or the fingertip in the same position. Hold for fifteen seconds. Release. Work in a circular pattern, covering the entire area.

POINTS 3 TO 4

- Locate the stress point along the line running out to the side of the shoulder.

- Use *direct pressure* on the spot, counting to fifteen. Release. Take your time and relax between strokes, remembering that this is a painful spot.

- Repeat the stroke. Increase the hold to twenty. Release. Wait a minute.

- Repeat one more time, counting to twenty. Release.

- Change to crossfiber *friction*. Hold for a count of fifteen. Release. Wait.

- Repeat the stroke, increasing the time you hold the point to twenty. Release.

- Repeat the stroke one more time. Count to twenty. Release.

POINT 4

- Locate the teres point on the lower outer shoulder.

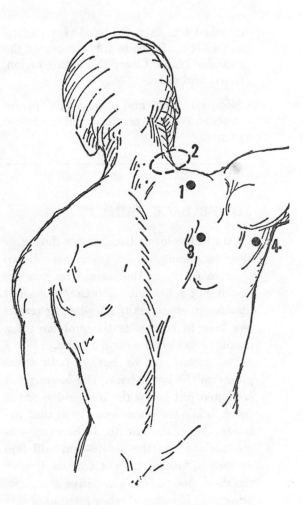

- Approaching the point from a side angle, apply *direct pressure* with the thumbtip penetrating the heavy muscle tissue. Hold for a count of fifteen. Release.

- Repeat the stroke, increasing the count to twenty. Release.

- Repeat one more time. Hold for twenty-five. Release.

- Change over to crossfiber *friction*. Hold for a count of twenty, working as deep as is comfortable. Release.

- Repeat the stroke twice, extending it to thirty seconds. Release.

POINT 5

- Finish off with a series of *compressions*, using the flat of the hand or a loosely clenched fist. Keep the hand very relaxed so that it conforms to the contour of the shoulder blade. Cover the entire region, slowly and steadily.

• Now go back and repeat the earlier strokes of *direct pressure* and crossfiber *friction*.

• Give further *compressions*.

• Repeat these sequences for a total of about twenty minutes the first time around.

LOWER BACK PAIN

Pain in the lower back, either during or after swimming, stems from one of two pressure points in that area. You can get on-the-spot relief with Sportsmassage, but in order to effect really long-lasting results you have to keep after the problem for a couple of weeks on a regular basis.

The spasm can be felt at both stress points on the lower back. The lower point is located just below the bony ridge of the pelvis, while the upper one lies against the lower edge of the last rib. In between—immediately above the pelvis—you will find an area of spasm. Do not confuse it with the stress points. It is a sensitive area, covering the kidneys and other internal organs with very little bony or muscular protection. Reserve your heavy work for the points themselves.

Direct pressure combined with crossfiber *friction* are used on the top points. Work with the thumb and fingertip. Follow up with a series of *compressions*, covering the entire buttock with three passes—palm of hand, heel of hand, and loosely clenched fist.

Then go back and reapply *pressure* and *friction*. The back will be much less painful. Repeat the three sequences a few more times—say, for a total of twenty or thirty minutes—and call it a day. Repeat the procedure again in a day or so and keep on with it regularly until the problem is cleared up.

EXERCISE:

The first exercises performed are actually tests to see how large a range of free motion has been created by the treatment. Ask the swimmer to turn over and bend his knees, keeping the feet flat on the floor. Then have him perform a series of bridging motions, raising the midsection as high as possible.

Have him get up and walk. Then do a series of deep knee bends. Finally, a few forward and backward bends. Take care that the forward bend is not performed without a hand support just in case the muscle grabs.

Regardless of how much better the situation, straight-legged toe touches are out. So are situps. People with chronic back problems should realize that situps are a cause of continued problems in this area, and they should seek an alternate form of stomach-tightening exercise.

Lower Back Pain

POINTS 1 AND 2

- Apply *direct pressure* with thumb or forefinger to each point in turn. Hold for a count of fifteen. Release.

- Repeat the stroke, increasing the time to twenty-five seconds. Release.

- Repeat once more. Hold to a count of thirty seconds. Release.

- Switch to crossfiber *friction*. Hold for a count of twenty. Release.

- Repeat the stroke for a count of thirty. Release.

- Repeat the same stroke once more.

POINT 3

- Use the palm of your hand to perform a slow, steady series of *compressions* over the entire area of the buttock.

- Repeat the series, this time using the heel of the hand.

- Finish up with another pass of *compressions*, using the fist loosely clenched.

- You cannot go back to try out the *pressure-friction* strokes once again. The pain will have lessened, but not disappeared totally.

- Work for another twenty minutes or so, no more, at this first session.

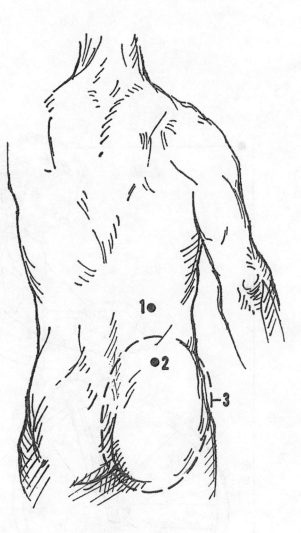

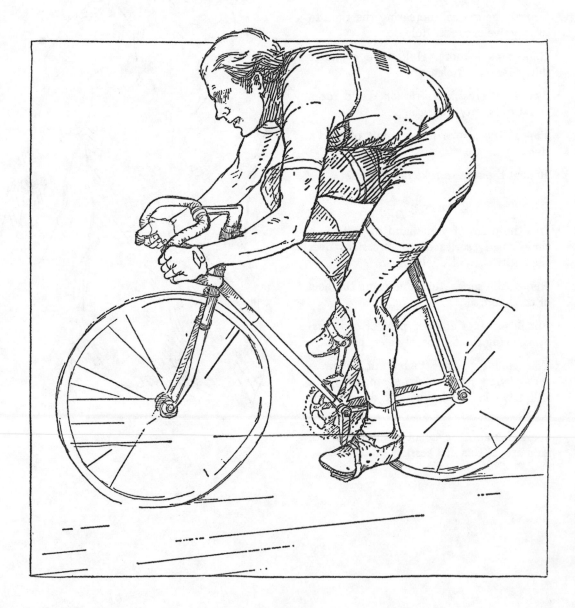

Cycling concentrates its stress on a minimum of body area. The legs, of course, are the prime breakdown areas, with muscle tightening and muscle fatigue forming the barrier that inhibits your continuing on with the race.

The Sore Points

Besides the legs, trouble spots occur in the lower back and shoulder area as well as in the forearms and hands. Due to the hunched-forward posture of distance cycling, the positions of those parts of the body are under an almost constant isometric type of strain that eventually leads to muscle fatigue.

When muscle fatigue hits, you feel it all over. Shoulders and back ache, which is an aggravation but no real threat to your finishing your ride or event. The hands and forearms, however, are another matter. Fatigue here can affect your control of the bicycle, and a cramp in a tight spot could be dangerous.

The overuse of the legs leads to fade, the inability to continue, or the onset of severe cramping. In the underconditioned cyclist,

weakness will signal the end of the event, while in the well-conditioned rider, tightening and loss of co-ordination are the nemeses.

For competitors, Sportsmassage will increase the time that any given pace can be maintained, will insure faster recuperation from problems, and will loosen the trouble spots against possible spasms during an arduous event. One of the best tests possible for the 20 per cent extra factor comes from amateur cyclists competing in a marathon. You feel—and use—the additional time and ease instantly.

WRIST STRAIN

When the wrist is held in forced hyperextension at the same time that the fist is clenched—in other words, the position in which you grip the handlebars—stress occurs. It occurs at the points where the muscles become interspersed with tendonous fibers at the wrist. The muscles responsible for flexing the forearm tighten, placing more stress upon the wrist attachments. You feel irritation and pain there, but until you press on the area you will be unaware of the actual spasms.

Pain can develop in any one of the six stress points, in the wrist area or it can be generalized. Treatment depends on the case. If it's individualized, concentrate on that spot. If it's general, do the whole set of points.

Direct pressure and crossfiber *friction* are used on the point or points themselves. Second, a general crossfiber *friction* is given to the wrist.

The entire forearm is gone over with deep, steady *compressions,* and the stress point or points get additional *direct pressure* as a finale.

EXERCISE:

Flexing the wrist and clenching the fist while the wrist is in flexion are the first exercises advisable. No stretching at all at this point.

After the pain has disappeared, gradual stretching can begin. On the matter of pain in cycling, you might note that the pain that develops in the back or the wrist from cycling is a result of a compression, or jamming effect. It occurs in the ligaments rather than in the tendons or muscles. To escape wrist tension, cyclists lower the handlebars—a good idea, but it tends to place the stress of the sport on the backs of the shoulders or the lower back itself.

Wrist Strain

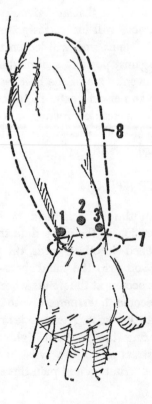

POINT 1, 2, 3, 4, 5, OR 6

- With your fingertips, probe to discover the seat of the spasm. It will feel stiff and tender to the touch.

- Apply *direct pressure* to the point. Hold for a count of fifteen. Release.

- Reapply the stroke, increasing the press to a count of twenty. Release.

- Repeat the stroke once again.

- Change to crossfiber *friction.* Work steadily and thoroughly for a count of twenty. Release.

- Reapply *friction,* again for a count of twenty. Release.

POINT 7

- Move on to the wrist itself. Have the player sit with the arm resting on a flat surface.

- Using the thumb, apply a steady crossfiber *friction* all around the wrist, front and back. Work steadily, slowly, and deeply. Hold each point for a count of twenty, then move on.

• Repeat the circle two more times.

POINT 8

• With the flat of your hand, begin a series of *compressions,* working up the entire forearm, front and back, from the wrist to the elbow. Work slowly and deeply, trying to spread the fibers out beneath the skin.

• Repeat the *compressions,* using the heel of the hand.

POINT 1, 2, 3, 4, 5, OR 6

• Finish up with a further application of *direct pressure* on the point or points in spasm. Press steadily and hold for a count of twenty. Release.

• Repeat the stroke.

• Make one more application, increasing the count of the hold to thirty. Release.

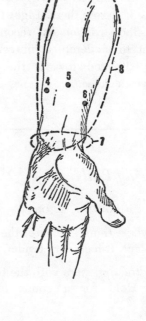

HAMSTRING PULLS

The thigh muscles of the cyclist are particularly susceptible to hamstring problems due to the action of cycling itself. It requires a continual shortening of the hamstrings with no lengthening balance. An offset exercise of stretching these muscles out regularly helps a good deal, but it is still a heavy area.

To determine which of the three possible stress points is involved in a hamstring situation, you have to apply pressure, which leaves little room for doubt. Beneath the point and extending downward to the midthigh region, you can feel a tight line of muscle.

If, however, the pain is felt in the lower third of the muscle extending down to the back of the knee, you have another, more difficult kind of hamstring to deal with. These points do not respond as readily to treatment and, being in the knee region,

are far more liable to recurrence and irritation.

Apply *direct pressure* and crossfiber *friction* to the upper stress points. *Compress* and *knead* the back of the thigh, gently and firmly grasping the cramped area and pulling it out to the side.

Depending upon the origin of the major stress, you will find a heavy line of spasm located in the upper portion of the muscle. Work on this with fist *compressions* and crossfiber *friction.*

When it is the lower portion of the hamstring that is injured, the stress points are found below the knee, most likely on the outer side. They are extremely tender. Use only the lightest pressure here, even less than used on the upper hamstring treatment. *Direct pressure* and crossfiber *friction* are used here.

Attention should be given to the back of the knee as well, particularly to the tendons passing across there. Light to moderate crossfiber *friction* is recommended; then light to moderate *compressions* and *kneading* directed toward the cramped area above the knee.

EXERCISE:

Attempt no stretches right away. The goal is to restore motion without aggravation, and in order to achieve that, you first have to achieve walking without pain, jogging, and running in the same fashion. After that you can go on to a fuller exercise regimen.

Hamstring Pull

POINT 1, 2, OR 3

- With your thumb, locate the primary stress point. It feels very tender.

- Apply *direct pressure* with the thumb. Be gentle. Hold for a count of fifteen. Release.

- Repeat the *pressure*, holding for a count of twenty. Release.

- Change to crossfiber *friction*. Work very gently, never beyond the point of tolerance. Hold for a count of twenty. Then release.

- Repeat the stroke. Hold to twenty-five. Release.

- Apply one more *friction*. Count to thirty. Then release.

POINT 4

- Apply a series of *compressions* with the flat of your hand. Work slowly and gently over the entire back of the thigh. Work down, from the buttocks to the knee.

- *Knead* the same area. Grasp the flesh firmly but gently. Pull it sideways with each stroke.

POINT 5

- Locate the thick line of spasm muscle running down four or five inches below the stress point here.

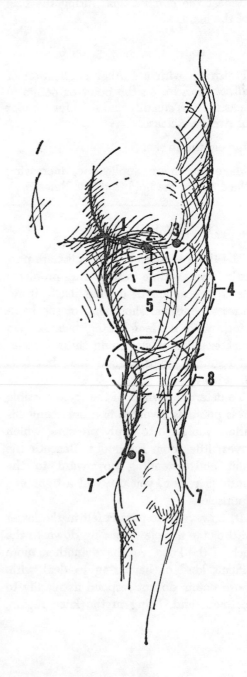

- Apply a series of fist *compressions* to the area. Work gently.

- Change to crossfiber *friction,* using the ends of the fingers. Cover the same area.

- *Now go back and rework the entire sequence of strokes, from the stress points on down.* Increase the pressure somewhat, but not beyond tolerance.

- Repeat the entire sequence one more time. Again, be firm, but do not stress the area further.

POINT 6

- Find the stress point on the lower part of the hamstring.

- Apply *direct pressure* with the thumb, holding for a count of fifteen. Release. *Be very careful, as this is an extremely sensitive area.*

- Repeat the stroke. Hold for twenty. Release.

- Repeat the stroke. Hold for twenty-five. Release.

- Apply crossfiber *friction* gently. Hold for a count of twenty. Release.

- Repeat the same gentle *friction* for a count of twenty-five. Release.

- Apply *friction* once more. Hold to thirty. Release.

POINT 7

- Locate with your fingertips the tendons from the hamstring passing down over the back of the knee.

- Apply a light, crossfiber *friction.* Count to twenty. Release.

- Work over the same area once again. Increase to a hold of thirty. Release.

POINT 8

- With your fingertips, locate the cramped area above the back of the knee.

- With the heel of the hand, apply a series of light to moderate *compressions.* Cover the entire region slowly and thoroughly.

- *Knead* the same area. Take care to give as much firmness as can be tolerated, but no more.

- Repeat both sequences one more time.

LOWER BACK PAIN

This is another of those spots where a few seconds of pressure can bring dramatic relief. But since the origin of the problem is connected with one of the inherent movements of the sport—forward bending —it's difficult to remove on a permanent basis.

The spasm is readily felt at both stress points on the lower back and is quite sensitive to pressure, as you will find out once you give it a probe with your finger. The upper point is just below and lying against the lower edge of the last rib. The lower one is located just below the bony ridge of the pelvis.

Immediately above the pelvic crest is an area of stiff spasm. Watch out for it! You are now over the kidney area, and there is no bony protection for the organs beneath. *It is an area that is never handled roughly, and under no circumstances ever given any* percussion *treatment.*

You will also find a good degree of tightening in the buttock region; give ample attention to that area as well.

There are two parts to the Sportsmassage technique for lower back trouble: direct work on the stress points and general massage for the buttocks. A combination of *direct pressure* and crossfiber *friction* is used in the first instance, a triple series of *compression* strokes in the second.

Once lightly through both sequences, repeat them, several times over perhaps. As they are reapplied, the back region becomes noticeably less painful. But it will never reach the point of causing no pain in this case, so don't push for it! You will overdo it if you keep on for too long.

EXERCISE:

Lie on your back and bend your knees, keeping your feet flat on the table. Raise your midsection as high as possible.

Then get up and test out the extent of restoration of movement: first by walking, then with a series of deep knee bends, and finally with gradual bending—forward and backward. *The forward bend is never done without a hand support just in case the muscle grabs.*

Regardless of how much improved the situation, it's not a good idea to try any straight-legged toe touches. People whose chronic back problems are centered in this section will find that doing situps is a cause of continued problems. If you need to tighten up your stomach muscles, better find another exercise.

Lower Back Pain

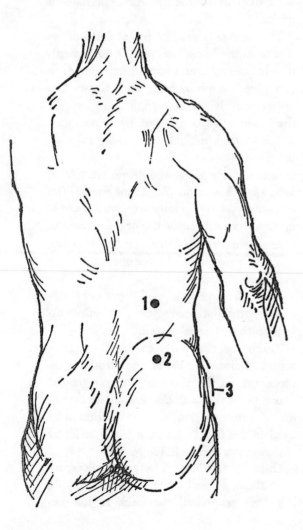

POINTS 1 AND 2

- Using your thumb or forefinger, apply *direct pressure* to the spot. Hold for a count of fifteen. Release.

- Reapply, increasing the hold to twenty-five. Release.

- Apply *pressure* one more time. Hold for a count of thirty. Release.

- Switch to crossfiber *friction*. Hold for a count of twenty. Release.

- Repeat the stroke for a count of thirty. Release.

- Repeat the same stroke.

POINT 3

- Using the palm of your hand, begin a slow, solid series of *compressions* that cover the entire area of the buttock.

- Repeat the series, using this time the heel of your hand.

- Repeat the series, switching to loosely clenched fists for the *compressions*.

- You can now go back and repeat the sequences in order again—*direct pressure*, crossfiber *friction*, and *compressions*, with pressure somewhat increased. Work for up to twenty or thirty minutes' total, then stop. That's enough for one session.

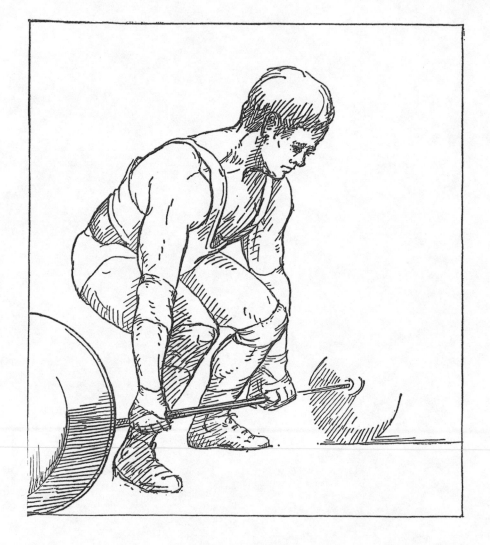

WEIGHT LIFTING AND BODY BUILDING

It was not too many years ago that weight lifting was universally frowned upon by coaches, trainers, and team physicians alike. Times have changed, and today weight training enjoys a degree of repute as great as its former disrepute.

The traditional disclaimers ran something like: "Weight lifting makes you musclebound, destroys your co-ordination, slows you down." Yet in spite of it all, athletes in ever-increasing numbers turned to weights in secrecy to boost their strength and performance quotients. I for one still remember the shock reflected when Cleveland fireball ace Bob Feller disclosed in a newspaper article that he had been lifting weights since a boy and had continued throughout his fabulous career. But even this disclosure came only after his retirement and then in a tone that was half apologetic and half defiant.

Football, a game that requires great strength, body bulk, and quickness, had the greatest influence upon the acceptance of weight training. It was here that men built their bodies up to tremendous size and strength through the ingestion of food and the handling of heavy weights and did it without sacrificing mobility and speed.

This success rapidly spread into every sport until today there are very few serious athletes who do not include some form of weight training in their programs. *There is no faster way to increase strength than with weights.*

Styles of Weight Lifting

The most important difference between the athletes who make the lifting of heavy weights their main concern and those who train with weights in order to gain increased strength for other fields of sports is the inclusion of flexibility exercises. Whereas the serious weight lifter puts between 90 and 100 per cent of his training into lifting, the other athlete will put in at least two hours of speed and flexibility training for every one hour spent on strength exercise. This is necessary to maintain mobility. Each does what he must do to excel at his chosen sport.

It is obvious when you watch the movements of the person who does nothing but lift heavy weights that he had to sacrifice a great deal of his mobility in order to build a platform capable of hoisting and holding tremendous poundages overhead. There are many football players who will match bench presses with high-level weight lifters, but in the overhead work—the press, clean and jerk, and snatch—they will be left behind, because this kind of work takes a certain degree of inflexibility, a certain thickening of the muscle fibers, the tendons, and the ligaments; and football players are too mobile for that.

The same distinction holds true between the Olympic-style weight lifter and the body builder who works equally hard. The American and the English schools of body building call for fully developed arms, legs, and upper torso, then a small waist and buttocks. While this group has the arm and leg strength to lift heavy weights aloft, the relatively small and flexible midsection will not support that same weight in an overhead position.

Thus that which is a strength aesthetically is a weakness structurally. And it is interesting to note that the classic Greco-Roman school of body culture considered this tiny waist a weakness and strove for the wider waist as its ideal.

The Basic Tenets of Weight Lifting

There are two basic tenets in weight lifting that are paramount whatever your style and purpose. *Heavy weights and low repetitions increase muscle size and strength. Lighter weights and high repetitions increase definition.*

Everything that is done ties in directly to those two simple facts of weight-lifting life. The Olympic-style lifter is not interested in well-defined muscles. His one and only aim is to raise the most possible weight to the overhead position. Most of his workouts are devoted to technique and strength-building exercise. Of all lifters he undergoes the greatest stress and strain.

The body builder is interested in symmetry, in enlarging certain muscle groups and leaving others undeveloped. He therefore employs alternate periods of heavy weight training for specific muscle groups coupled with a high-calorie diet and high repetitions with lower weights and lower calories to mark definitions in the muscles.

Trouble Spots

The greatest number of strain-type injuries occur to the Olympic weight lifters. Also the greatest number of more serious injuries. It is not uncommon for a knee or an ankle to collapse under the intense pressure placed upon it.

Many years ago I was acquainted with Dave Mayer in Philadelphia. Dave won the gold medal in the 1936 Olympics with a press of 376 pounds. But his career ended on a routine working day when his hip collapsed while he was holding 250 pounds overhead during a regular training session!

The most common problems encountered by Olympic lifters are *strains in the upper shoulder and base of the neck*. These strains occur at the point of the lift as the arms start to come up. Complete discussion for treatment of this type of injury is included in the baseball chapter.

Lower down the arm, *the triceps* comes in for its share of strain, with most of the pain being felt in the elbow joint. This aggravation comes from the locking out at the top of either the snatch or the clean and jerk.

Lower back pain is related to strain at the very beginning of the lift. It is further aggravated by the tightening of the muscles while getting the weight up to the fully raised position. Interesting enough, the therapy for this kind of strain is closely related to that for lower back trouble in skiing. See that section of the book for full details on handling it.

Last but not least by any stretch of the imagination is the *strain placed on the legs, particularly on the outside of the lower thigh muscles.* Pain here is generally most intense near the knee joint. This occurs at the very beginning point of the lift. See the section on skiing for a full account of Sportsmassage for this area.

Body builders have many more shoulder problems than Olympic lifters because of the different style of training. One of the main viewing features, the chest, requires a lot of heavy bench pressing to enlarge the pectorals.

The first strain occurs in the tissue at the breastbone and is followed by spasms in the pectoral muscle itself. You also feel pain when you raise your arm sideways. Here the original strain occurs at the bottom of the bench press and is aggravated with usage.

Triceps strain for this type of weight training is more apt to be in the belly of the muscle and to come about as a result of repetitions rather than at the end when locking out.

The source of lower back pain for the body builder is usually slightly different than with the weight lifter. Use of the quadriceps machine to enlarge the front of the thighs means fewer of the tremendous number of squats usually done by Olympic lifters. The body builder also does much more bending, twisting, and situps. The strains come more from rotating and bending. And again, treatment for trouble in this area is fully covered in the chapter on skiing.

PRO TIP

On training young athletes with the use of weights, this sports era places intense pressure upon youngsters to increase muscle size and strength rapidly, perhaps too rapidly for accommodation by the body. On any given day at the Y, kids come up to me to ask about this pain or that pain. These are teen-agers in their full resiliency, people for whom muscle injury should be very rare.

Almost invariably these problems are connected with overdone weight training for their sport. Because it has been so successful, nothing is going to change it, but something is being lost along the way when young bodies are forced to the limit at such an early stage in their career.

So this is what I tell any coach who asks me about weight training. If you are breaking a newcomer into weight lifting, the first thing a youngster is going to do is see how much he can lift. You're not going to stop him. It's the nature of the young beast.

But you might contain him by pointing out how a strain or more serious injury will retard his ultimate progress. Give him a timetable he can live with. Say, "Do what I tell you for three months and then you can go for max." It usually works and you've given the youngster just that much more of a head start on properly preparing his body for maximum strain than he would have had if left on his own.

SHOULDER/CHEST PAIN

A common site of deltoid (upper arm) strain is just below the rounded portion of that muscle, front, back, or middle. From the stress point, you'll feel a tight line running up to the tip of the shoulder. The culprit is likely to be either lateral dumbbell raises or wide grip presses behind the neck.

Treatment is a combination of *direct pressure* and crossfiber *friction* applied to the sore portion of the muscle. Follow this up with *compressions*, working over the entire muscle good and deep. After that initial softening up, you can move in with further crossfiber *frictions* directly on the line of tightness all the way up to the shoulder tip. Follow that with another application of *direct pressure* to the stress point itself.

EXERCISE:

A simple exercise to follow up the above routine is performed by pressing up against the top of a doorframe. That's it. No lateral raises should be attempted at this time.

Also very common among weight lifters is the pain that occurs as the arm comes forward from an extreme backward position—the bottom of the bench press with maximum weight. The spasm develops in the collarbone portion of the chest muscle and pain shoots out toward the shoulder.

Closer inspection and a good deal of sharp poking around reveal two distinct, painful areas. One is where the chest muscle meets the breastbone. The other, which feels like a nodule, is found just below the collarbone about halfway between the breastbone and the tip of the shoulder.

Direct pressure and crossfiber *friction* directly on this collarbone point start off the treatment. This is a very painful point, so use less pressure for longer periods and do more sequences. Press *this point only once for thirty seconds only*. Overwork here can cause an onset of adverse symptoms. It is easily irritated.

For the breastbone area, a combination of *direct pressure* and crossfiber *friction* brings quick relief.

EXERCISE:

What you want at this time is a no-strain, full-contraction exercise. Press your hands together in an isometric fashion or press the hand of the affected side against the opposite shoulder. No vigorous backward movement should be performed at this time.

Shoulder and Chest Pain

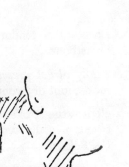

POINT 1, 2, OR 3

- Have the player sit facing a bench or table, forearms placed upon it for support.

- Locate the exact stress point with the tip of the thumb or forefinger. Apply *direct pressure*, holding for a count of fifteen. Release.

- Reapply the same stroke. Increase the pressure slightly and extend to twenty-five seconds. Release.

- Repeat the above stroke. Release.

- Switch to crossfiber *friction*. Hold for a count of twenty. Release.

- Repeat the *friction* twice more, each time increasing the pressure and extending the hold for five seconds.

POINT 4

- Begin a series of deep *compressions*, to cover the entire muscle. Work slowly and deeply, circling from the outside rim of the muscle toward the center.

POINT 5

- Using the point of the thumb, begin a sharp crossfiber *friction* to the tight line of muscle running up from the stress point to the tip of the shoulder. Work deeply and hold each *friction* for a count of fifteen. Then release and move up an inch or so toward the top of the shoulder.

- Now go back and apply *direct pressure* once again to the original stress point. Hold for a count of twenty. Release.

- Repeat twice more.

POINT 6

- Apply *direct pressure* to the point on the collarbone. Keep it light and hold for a count of thirty. Release. *Do no more work here at this session.*

- Further sequences of *pressure* can be performed on the breastbone point from time to time over a period of several days. But keep the pressure light. Work on the collarbone point no more than once a day for no more than thirty seconds at a time.

POINT 7

- Have the player change to a face-lying-up position with hands at sides.

- Locate the tender stress point on the breastbone.

- Apply *direct pressure* very lightly. Hold for a count of twenty. Release.

- Repeat the stroke, increasing the count to twenty-five, but varying the pressure little. Release.

- Repeat the stroke again, increasing the count to thirty. Release.

TRICEPS STRAIN

A couple of things can cause this particular strain. You diagnose which is which by the seat of the pain. If it is felt directly in the belly of the muscle, the source is generally an overuse in extension exercises. When it is felt in the elbow joint, it comes from a sudden violent motion, such as "locking out" a heavy clean and jerk.

The central pressure point is the same in either instance—about two inches above the elbow slightly outside the middle. It is a hot-coal kind of strain, and once you reach it, you have no trouble feeling the knot beneath the surface. Pressure tolerance for this point is very limited, so the general plan of attack is *less more often.*

A minute of *direct pressure* followed by a minute of crossfiber *friction* repeated ten or twelve times with a good rest between each session works best. In the in-between time you can give a series of deep *compressions* to the complete triceps, shoulder to elbow.

If the pain is referred to the elbow joint, you can add crossfiber *friction* across the top of the joint.

EXERCISE:

Try moderate to full contractions of the arm from an extended or nearly extended position. Don't try any full contractions from a fully flexed position at this time.

Triceps Strain

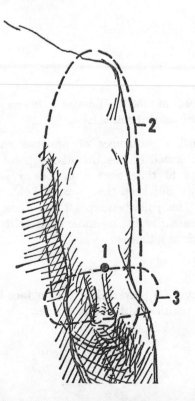

POINT 1

- Have the player sit or stand. Draw and support the arm backward with one of your hands placed at the front of the elbow. Use the other hand to massage.

- With thumb or fingertip apply *direct pressure* to the point. Hold for a count of twenty. Release. Remember to keep it gentle.

- Repeat the same stroke twice more. Keep the pressure light.

- Change to crossfiber *friction*. Hold for a count of twenty, working gently. Release.

- Repeat the *friction* twice more at the same pressure and rate.

- This two-part sequence can be repeated ten or twelve times with substantial rest periods in between.

POINT 2

- Begin a series of deep *compressions* using the palm of your hand or a loose fist. Work over the entire surface of the muscle from shoulder to elbow. Work deeply and steadily.

POINT 3

- If there is pain in the elbow, apply crossfiber *friction* across the top of the joint. Work as deeply as is comfortably possible. Hold each stroke for a count of fifteen. Then release. Work from inner to outer side.

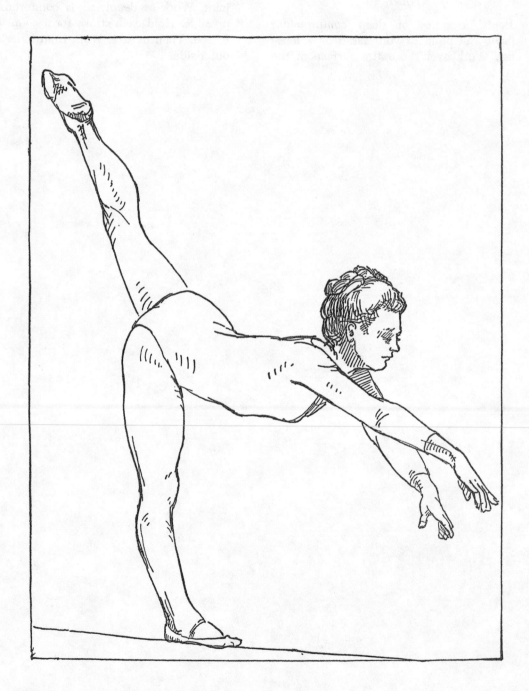

One reason I chose that Nureyev quote in the front of the book is that it really zeroes in on the critical factor that differentiates dance from most other types of sports activities. That is the constant, unavoidable strain.

Unlike many other physical endeavors, dance gives you no way out to change your stance when you are in a position of overstretch. When a performance calls on you to perform a certain movement in a certain prescribed manner, it must be done regardless of the pain involved.

In so many sports, you can protect the tiny ache and pain. If it's bothering you to go straight in, for example, you can turn your body slightly. You can't do that in dancing because it is a precision routine.

You start out with maybe a slight nagging in the shoulder. At first it's not obvious, until you start to cool down. Then you start to feel it when you get up in the morning. But after you work a little, the trouble clears up. For a while.

But eventually you reach the point where the pain doesn't disappear in your warmup. Now you make one wrong move one day—twisting, turning, catching your partner—and wham! You get the blinding stab. You have to start bracing yourself to get into a different position, and of course it shows. Eventually that support wears away and the severe injury occurs. You've had it for a week or two!

Trouble Spots

It virtually goes without saying that dancing has an almost unlimited potential for causing problems due to the wide variety of movements herded together under that one category. How you strain or hurt yourself, naturally, depends upon how you dance. But one obvious factor in dancing is that many of the movements most valued by performer and audience alike rely on gravity- and balance-defying postures that stress the body to the nth degree.

Any form of dance that involves lifting a partner about—be it ballet or Apache dancing—puts a severe strain on *the neck and shoulders* of the lifting partner. Therefore I am not being facetious when I suggest that if this applies to you, you would do well to take a look at the chapter on weight lifting, with special reference to the strokes and check points for the shoulders and upper back.

Also, *hamstrings*. Overstress of the thigh muscles is an easy mark for a dancer. A routine self-check for the stress points in this area can save a lot of wear and tear on the legs. The section on basketball covers this pretty thoroughly later in the book.

The last major area that gets a thorough workout in dancing is the *lower back and hips*. Many forms of dance or individual dance steps require a hypertension to be maintained in this region. This puts a constant stress on *the pelvis and the upper thigh muscles*. Your strongest power position is having the pelvis rolled slightly forward. Rolled backward—a stance commonly assumed in dancing—is one of the weakest and places great stress on the surrounding parts of the body, which then must compensate for the loss.

LOWER BACK STRESS

It's an easy matter to locate the two stress points on the lower back. They're sensitive to pressure. The top one is found just below the lower edge of the last rib. The bottom one is just below the bony ridge of the pelvis.

Start off with *direct pressure* and crossfiber *friction*. The first time around, both points will be extremely pressure-sensitive. So then try a change of tactics and do some general *compression* work on the whole buttock region. Afterward, go back to the stress points and give them some more attention.

Keep up this alternating between stress points and buttock several times over. The points will relax considerably, but not completely in just one sitting. So keep on massaging them at regular intervals over the next week.

EXERCISE:

Ask the dancer to turn over on his back and to bend his knees, keeping his feet flat on the table. Ask him to make a bridge, raising the midsection up as high as possible. Tell him to relax and try it again. Repeat this a few more times.

Then have him get up and walk around a bit. Try a series of deep knee bends, and, finally, some gradual bending, backward and forward. Don't let him try the forward bend without some sort of hand support—in case the muscle should grab. That's about it. And remember—*no situps!*

Lower Back Stress

POINTS 1 AND 2

• Have the dancer lie face down on a table.

• Locate the stress point with your thumb or forefinger.

• Apply *direct pressure* for a count of fifteen. Release.

• Repeat the stroke, increasing the hold to twenty-five. Release.

• Repeat the stroke. Hold for a count of thirty. Release.

• Change the stroke to crossfiber *friction*. Hold for a count of twenty. Release.

• Repeat the stroke, increasing the hold to a count of thirty. Release.

• Repeat the same stroke.

POINT 3

• Use the palm of your hand to do a series of solid *compressions* covering the entire area of the buttock.

• Repeat the *compressions*, using the heel of the hand.

• Repeat the series, using a loosely clenched fist.

• You can now go back to work on the stress points again, then a series of *compressions*. Work like this, alternating strokes, for a total of twenty to thirty minutes.

PAIN IN HIP AREA

The high frequency of trunk twists and bends in dancing makes it a sport ripe for lower back and hip troubles. The section following takes on the whole lot of them, more than you will probably have at any one time. But, nevertheless, it is always a safe idea to check these points out on your-

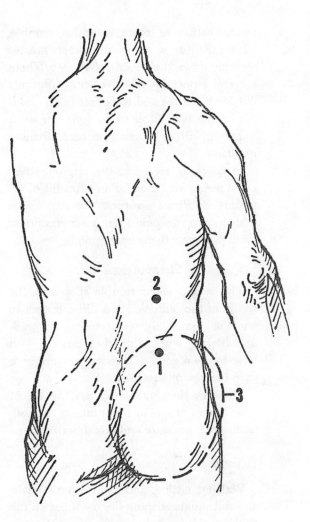

self, if only as a matter of preventive maintenance.

So choose and pick which of the following pain points apply to you. And save the rest for future reference. They fall into three general categories.

Stress Area One

This point is located on the extreme outside of the hip, generating tightening and pain all the way down the leg and up into the lower back. *Direct pressure* and crossfiber *friction* directly on the point begin the treatment.

If you feel pain going down your leg, it's

an indication of more extensive trouble. This calls for a series of *direct presses* working down the outside of the leg. There are two especially sensitive spots—one just outside the knee and the other in the middle of the calf. Stop to perform an extra minute of *direct pressure* on each of these points.

In between, return to the original stress point five or six times for an extra bit of attention via *direct pressure*. You will notice a sharp drop in pain after your second or third pass over the original point.

Stress Area Two

The second major trouble spot is in the center of the buttock. It's a difficult area to work on, especially on persons with well-upholstered rears. For that reason, you have to use a good deal more pressure here than in most other areas.

To work the point well, use the tip of your thumb or one or more fingers, braced, with *direct pressure* and crossfiber *friction*.

EXERCISE:

Walking, sitting, and rising from a chair, and full squats keeping the heels flat on the floor are the lead-off exercises for this area.

Do only enough squats to establish painless motion, no more.

Stress Area Three

This point is found on the side of the hip just an inch or so away from the first one mentioned in this section. It feels like a tight cramp running around the side of the hip down toward the groin area. Even though you may at first think that the pain is centered in the lower back, a little work on this spot makes you realize that it is coming from one side of the hip.

Both *direct pressure* and crossfiber *friction* should be applied to the point. However, use less pressure overall than in other areas—you're dealing with a wider mass of muscle.

In contrast, you use full deep *pressure* on the spasm line that runs down to the head of the thighbone. Otherwise you won't make a dent in it.

EXERCISE:

The best exercise is a simple trunk twist from a seated position. Then a trunk twist from a standing position, drawing your knee up toward your chest as though putting on a sock. Avoid situps.

Pain in Hip Area

POINT 1

- Have the dancer lie face down, legs out in back as straight as possible. If tense, the sore leg can be crossed over the other leg at the ankle.

- Locate the pressure point at the outside of the hip.

- Using the thumb, apply *direct pressure* for a count of fifteen. Release. You may find that approaching the point from the side gives you better contact.

- Repeat the stroke. Increase to twenty. Release.

- Repeat the stroke. Increase the count to twenty-five. Release.

- Switch to crossfiber *friction*. Hold for fifteen seconds. Release.

- Repeat the stroke, increasing the time held to twenty. Release.

- Repeat the stroke again. Hold for a count of twenty-five. Release.

- Come back to this stress point five or six times during the rest of the session with additional *direct pressure*. You will notice that the sensitivity decreases with each new approach.

POINT 2

- Go on with *direct pressure* with the thumb working down the outside line of the leg. Hold each point for a count of ten. Then release and move an inch on down.

- You will find two tender points along the way.

POINT 3

- The first of these points is on the outside of the knee.

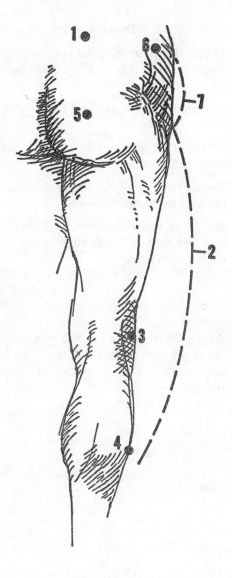

- Apply another minute of *direct pressure* here—fifteen-second presses with pauses in between.

POINT 4

- The second stress point is in the middle of the side of the calf. Apply *direct pressure* in the same manner—fifteen-second presses alternated with rest breaks.

Point 5

- Locate this pressure point—in the middle of the buttock. It feels like a tight ball or a mass of strings.

- Apply deep *direct pressure* for a count of fifteen. Release.

- Change to crossfiber *friction*. Hold for a count of fifteen. Release.

- Repeat the stroke, increasing the time of the hold to twenty. Release.

- Return to this point with additional *direct pressure* several more times. Go deeper each time.

Point 6

- Apply *direct pressure* to this point, using either the thumb or the tips of the four fingers. Hold for a count of fifteen. Release.

- Repeat the stroke, increasing the hold to twenty. Release.

- Go on to crossfiber *friction*. Hold for a count of fifteen. Release.

- Repeat the *friction*. Increase the holding time to twenty. Release.

- Return to this point again before finishing up. It is better to make more passes using less pressure in this area.

Point 7

- Locate the tight line running down from the previous point.

- Apply full *direct pressure* with the point of the thumb. Hold for a count of fifteen. Release.

- Increase the time of the stroke to twenty, repeating it.

- Continue to apply deep *direct pressure* down the length of the spasm.

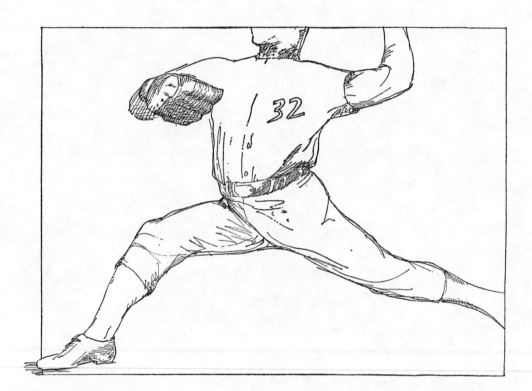

The game of baseball is comprised of so many different, specialized movements that it's not easy to pick out any typical problems that relate to all players of the game. But since everyone has to throw the ball at one time or another, we'll start with that basic motion—pitching.

Pitchers are notorious for having "bad arms." In reality, a major portion of the arm trouble has its source elsewhere—in the back, chest, or shoulder in most cases. In fact, it's a pretty safe bet that that mysterious arm trouble can be directly traced to one or another specific muscle group, depending upon the style of pitching you favor.

An overhand thrower, for instance, is more apt to run into difficulty with the longissimus dorsi lying under the shoulder, while a three-quarter or sidearm thrower can generally seek his source farther up in the trapezius and teres muscles of the upper back.

And for all pitchers, the pectorals of the upper chest are prime causes of stiffness and restricted motion. A cramp here can easily debilitate the rest of your body insofar as power and co-ordination go. It's a red-line area for a pregame check if you demand of your body speed and control at a moment's notice.

The other major area as far as pitching goes is the stomach, or abdomen. Under pressure or fatigue, these muscles are a potent source of tightening. A pitcher must have total movement in the midsection or else he is playing under an almost insurmountable handicap.

We certainly don't want to neglect batters in this discussion of baseball problems. Like the pitcher, the batter finds the neck, shoulder, and upper back region a hotbed of potential trouble spots.

Any restriction here—whether from tension, fatigue, or injury—holds up the total fluidity of the swing. Batting demands instantaneous reflexes. Remember that what you have are two rounded surfaces—the ball and the bat—coming together for a fraction of a second at a high rate of speed. To connect at all is some sort of small miracle. To put all you've got behind that connection is another one on a larger scale.

TIGHT CHEST

The cause of this difficulty is an abuse suffered during a variation of Basic Movement No. 11, arms-backward stretch. As the arm comes forward, rolling up and over the shoulder, you feel the strain, and pain shoots out toward the end of the shoulder.

In fact, there are two distinct stress points involved here. One is at the point where the chest muscle meets the breastbone. The other, which will feel like a hard, unripe grape beneath your fingertip, is found right beneath the collarbone at about the midpoint.

Direct pressure and crossfiber *friction* are used on the collarbone point. Since it is very sensitive, it's a better idea to go easy on the pressure and work a little longer than usual to make up for it. You can also do more sequences. One *press* held for thirty seconds is enough per session.

For the breastbone stress point, an effective combination is *direct pressure* followed by crossfiber *friction*. This is a responsive point, and relief comes quickly.

EXERCISE:

A no-strain, full-contraction exercise is what is needed here. Try pressing your hands together firmly. Or press the hand of the affected side against the opposite shoulder for a minute or two. Attempt no vigorous backward movements at this time.

Tight Chest

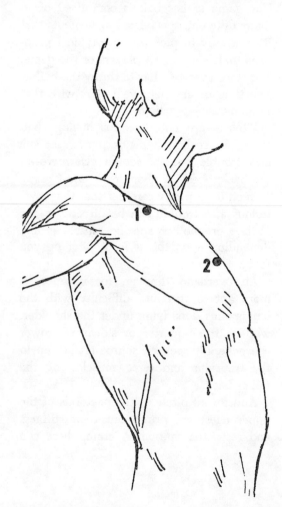

POINT 1

- Have the player lie face up with hands at the sides.

- Locate the stress point beneath the collarbone at its midpoint.

- Apply *direct pressure very lightly*. Hold for a count of thirty. Release. *Do no more work on this point this session.*

POINT 2

- Locate the stress point on the breastbone. Apply *direct pressure* lightly. Hold for a count of twenty. Release.

- Repeat the stroke, increasing the count to twenty-five, but keeping the pressure the same. Release.

- Repeat the stroke again. Increase the hold to a count of thirty. Release.

- Change your stroke to crossfiber *friction*. Hold for a count of twenty. Release.

- Repeat the stroke, increasing to a count of twenty-five. Release.

- Do one more *friction*, holding the press for a count of thirty. Then release.

- Further sequences can be performed over the next several days. Remember to do no more than one thirty-second press on the collarbone point per day.

UPPER BACK, SHOULDER PAIN

There are three trouble spots in the upper back region that trigger problems in the neck, shoulder, and high back regions. Two are connected to the shoulder blade itself—one at the top and one in the middle. The third point is located in the teres muscle, the bulge just beneath the arm where it connects to the back.

In the first instance, pain usually travels up—into the head and neck. You feel stiff and achy and even feel a sinus block on that side on occasion. Crossfiber *friction* directly on the stress point and also on the curve where the neck and shoulder join brings very fast relief here.

The midblade pain, which is actually seated in the midtrapezius, is a major spasm joint for any kind of heavy-duty shoulder work. It is also one of the most painful spots you can work on when it's in trauma. Here you feel pain shooting down into the arm, even tingling in the hand if the spasm is sufficiently severe.

What you concentrate on in this instance is the tight line you can feel running down at an angle from the midscapula to the stress point beneath the arm. It's not hard to find. It's very painful and feels tight as a banjo string. Give very gentle *direct pressure* and crossfiber *friction* with plenty of rest periods in between.

The teres stress point gets its own dose of *direct pressure* angled from the side to give better contact. This is followed by a session of crossfiber *friction* using a back-and-forth motion as you hook your thumb over the outer edge of the shoulder blade right there.

The final touch is an overall massage for the whole of the shoulder blade done with *compressions*.

EXERCISES:

Very simply, do some arm presses—backward and downward only. Do no forward or upward stretches right now.

Upper Back, Shoulder Pain

POINT 1

- Have the player lie face down, hands beneath the forehead.

- Apply crossfiber *friction* using the tip of the thumb or a braced finger. Hold for fifteen seconds. Release.

- Repeat the stroke. Hold for a count of twenty. Release.

- Repeat. Hold for a count of twenty-five. Release.

POINT 2

- If a stiff neck is present, work on the spot where the neck and shoulder join. Use crossfiber *friction.*

- Using the thumb or the fingertip held flat against the skin surface, work over the area in a circular fashion, holding each point for a count of fifteen, then releasing.

POINTS 3 TO 4

- Locate the stress point along the line running out to the side of the shoulder.

- Use *direct pressure*, counting to fifteen with each stroke. Take your time and relax in between strokes.

- Repeat the stroke. Increase the time to twenty seconds. Release. Rest.

- Repeat one more time. Count to twenty. Release.

- Change to crossfiber *friction.* Hold for a count of fifteen. Release. Pause.

- Repeat, increasing the time held to twenty. Release. Pause.

- Repeat one more time. Count to twenty. Release.

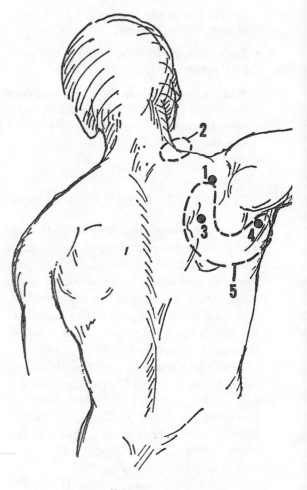

POINT 4

- Locate the teres point on the lower outer shoulder.

- Approach the point from the side. Apply *direct pressure* with the thumbtip. Hold for a count of fifteen. Release.

- Repeat the stroke. Increase the count to twenty. Release.

- Repeat once more. Hold for a count of twenty-five. Release.

- Change to crossfiber *friction.* Hold for a count of twenty, working as deeply as possible. Release.

• Repeat the stroke two more times. Extend the hold to thirty seconds. Release.

POINT 5

• Finish off with a series of *compressions*, using the flat of the hand or a loosely clenched fist. Keep your hand very relaxed to conform to the curve of the shoulder blade. Cover the whole area, working slowly, steadily, and deeply.

• Now go back to repeat the earlier strokes of *direct pressure* and crossfiber *friction*.

• Do more *compressions*.

• Work on these three sequences alternately for a total of about twenty minutes in the first session.

TENSED ABDOMEN

The stomach—abdomen for the purists —consists of three sets of muscles for twisting and turning (the obliques), and the rectus abdominis, running straight down the middle, for forward bending.

The common stress areas are the middle and lower attachments of the rectus, and on the sides, the points where the obliques attach to the crest of the pelvis. All these muscles get a workout in all total body movement either as prime movers or as maintainers of balance.

Treatment of the rectus is described in depth in the opening section on Sportsmassage. As for the obliques, you can find the stress points by running your fingers along the upper edge of the pelvis until you come to a tender spot. Crossfiber *friction* with the thumb or a braced finger loosens up the knot in a hurry.

PRO TIP

The rectus abdominis is one of the body's major points of tension. It goes rigid whenever the pressure pours on. An effective way to relax yourself whenever you feel yourself getting uptight is to directly manipulate the rectus.

Bend forward until you feel the muscle relax under your fingertips. Then press in toward the tightening from both sides with the points of the thumbs, compressing the muscle between them. Nature's tranquilizer!

Tensed Abdomen

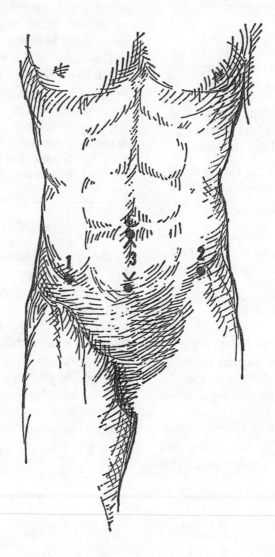

Point 1 or 2

- Have the player lie down facing up.

- Locate the tender spot on the pelvic crest.

- Using your thumb or a braced finger, apply crossfiber *friction*. Work as deeply as is comfortable. Hold for a count of twenty. Release.

- Repeat the stroke three more times. Hold each stroke for a count of twenty. Then release.

Point 3

- Follow the instructions in the general Sportsmassage for rectus abdominis or

- Give yourself the Pro Tip treatment mentioned above.

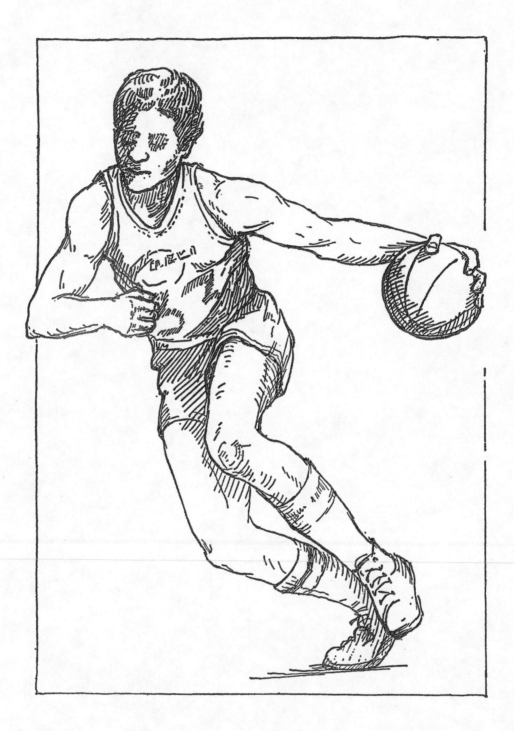

BASKETBALL

From the viewpoint of Sportsmassage, there are two things about the game of basketball that stand out: The game is played on a hard surface, and the game is played by big, exceptionally tall persons. As slender as most basketball players are, their weight is comparable with that of football players. And heavy weight coupled with hard surface means rough work for the ankle, knee, and hip joints.

The unusual length of the leg compounds the shock felt by the knee joint, so that many basketball players suffer a form of traumatic arthritis. Because of repeated shocks to this area and to the hip joints, there is a tendency toward tightening and loss of mobility throughout the hips and thighs. Quadriceps (thigh muscles) strains (commonly known as charley horses), hamstrings, and calf pulls all predominate as a result of this tightening.

Two other areas receive a hard going-over. The ankles, the base rotators of the body, take lots of punishment in this game, so you see scores of taped, strained, and sprained ankles both on the court and on the bench. Then there's the strain on the chest muscles caused by the upward arm-stretch movement characteristic of the game. Overstretch here can lead to spasms severe enough to lock a player's chest in its own iron cage, unable to relax, move, or breathe properly.

In fact, every stress point of the body gets a workout in basketball. But it's the legs that signal the end of a career. It's the premature onset of muscle tightening that costs the veteran performer that extra step.

It's the gap between the tiring of the self and the body. Everything else moves as it always did. The eye is still good. The hand is still quick. The rest of the body just has too much trouble getting where it has to be to make the play. Tiredness sets in sooner, and by the end of the game, the player is more and more apt to be caught out of position or late getting to his required slot. One slow player can throw off an entire team, and there is nothing left but to replace him with somebody younger who can keep up.

I don't think that very many players in basketball—or in any other sport, for that matter—ever really want to quit. Sports is a beautiful way of life. But when the exhaustion and the pressure of trying to keep up become too much, the smart player call it quits before the boobirds get to him.

Others, for various reasons, drag it out to the inevitable conclusion. All would continue longer if they could. And Sportsmassage can give them an extra two or three seasons, barring accident. For those who love the game, that extra time is a bonus in lifestyle as well as a financial remuneration.

CHEST LOCK

The seat of a chest-lock spasm is in the long, deep muscle that extends up the length of the back near the spine, the longissimus dorsi. Many movements can stress the point, but in the case of basketball, it is the overhead stretch with raised arms that signals the spasm. When that occurs, pain and lockage radiate into the front of the chest, causing breathing difficulty.

Sportsmassage here works down the back to the lower edge of the rib cage rather than upward toward the shoulder blade. Thumb *pressure* on the spasm itself is followed by crossfiber *friction*. The entire length of the muscle then receives both *compressions* and crossfiber *friction*. You should notice a painful area about four inches in length about halfway down. Extra *frictions* are in order here, as well as on the rhomboid muscles stretching from the upper spine to under the shoulder blade.

An appropriate follow-up exercise is pressing the arms backward and down. Do no forward or upward stretching at this time.

Chest Lock

POINT 1

- Have the player lie on his stomach with arms under the forehead.

- The stress point is located about 1½ inches below the inner, lower corner of the shoulder blade. It feels like a small nodule.

- Apply *direct pressure* with the thumb. Hold for a count of fifteen. Release.

- Repeat the stroke, holding for a count of twenty. Release.

- Apply one more *direct pressure*, increasing the time to thirty seconds. Release.

- Change to crossfiber *friction* using the thumb or braced finger. Hold for fifteen seconds. Release.

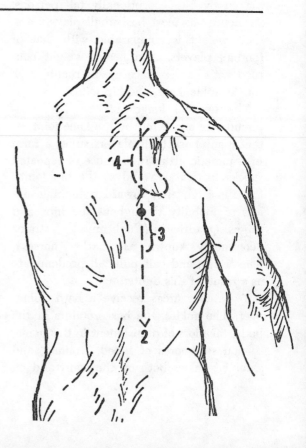

• Repeat the stroke. Hold for twenty-five seconds. Release.

POINT 2

• Using the flat of the hand, do a series of *compressions* down the length of the muscle. Work slowly and deeply.

• Change to the heel of the hand and repeat the *compression* sequence. Be firm.

• Do one more pass with the heel of the hand. Work in as deeply and as solidly as you can.

• Use your thumb to apply a deep crossfiber *friction* along the outer edge of the muscle. Take your time and work deeply.

POINT 3

• Give special attention to the sensitive area of the muscle—an area about 4 inches long in the middle of the muscle.

• Use the thumb to give additional deep crossfiber *frictions* here. Count to fifteen for each. Release.

• Repeat the sequence once more.

POINT 4

• Press your fingertips or thumbs deep into the furrow behind the shoulder blade.

• Apply a solid crossfiber *friction*. Work slowly and deeply. Count to fifteen. Release.

• Repeat the stroke. Increase to a count of twenty-five. Release.

SPRAINED ANKLE

Considering the beating the ankles take in the game of basketball, it's a wonder this problem doesn't crop up even more often than it does. But I suppose that basketball players, being aware of this particular weakness, pay closer attention to trouble in the ankle area than players in other sports and try to ward it off with such preventive techniques as ankle rolls or other exercises that strengthen the stress points here.

Any ankle injury demands quick attention. Get off the ankle and get somebody to take a look at it to determine just what has happened. Don't attempt any Sportsmassage or any other kind of manipulative therapy until it has had a chance to rest itself out. This can take up to a week, but it means the difference between further rupture injury and getting to work on the injury when the ankle is at maximum readiness to return to normal use.

With ankle injuries, you have to locate the adhesions by feel—very gentle feel. The original ruptures can have occurred anywhere, and you can only find them by gently moving the injured tissue with the tips of your fingers until you spot them.

Start out with a pass of crossfiber *friction* underneath the ankle joint, working over each of the sore spots. Move on to the instep where the ligaments and tendons are also in a state of stress and apply *friction*, first circular, then crossfiber.

On the outer side of the leg about three inches above the ankle is a very painful area. Here you use both *direct pressure* and crossfiber *friction* to bring relief.

The calf needs attention as well. There are always secondary lesions in this area and you cannot take the chance of neglecting them or you will never recover a full range of motion. A series of deep *compressions* covering the entire outside and back of the calf does the trick.

Sprained Ankle

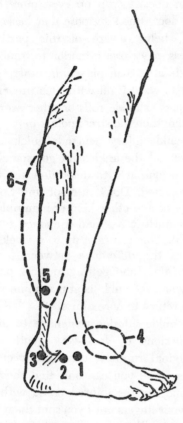

POINTS 1, 2, AND 3

- Have the player sit with the ankle out in front, supported from below.

- Apply crossfiber *friction* with the thumb or the forefinger. Be *very* gentle. Hold for a count of fifteen. Release.

POINT 4

- Place the heel of your hand on the base of the instep. Using gentle *friction*, massage up in slow, circular movements. Work up to the ankle, doing first the sides, then the middle of the instep. Count to ten for each stroke. Release.

- Go back to the base of the instep. With the flat of your thumb, apply crossfiber *friction*. Work for fifteen seconds. Release.

- Move up a little more. Reapply the *friction*. Work to fifteen. Release.

- Continue crossfiber *friction*. Work on the ligaments and tendons between the bones of the instep, slowly and deeply, all the way up to the ankle.

POINT 5

- Place the flat of your thumb on this point. Apply *direct pressure*. Hold for a count of fifteen. Release.

- Repeat twice more. Do not press any harder than is comfortable.

- Switch the stroke to crossfiber *friction*. Count to ten. Release.

- Do two more *frictions* at the same pace and pressure.

POINT 6

- For this stroke, the player must be lying face down. If working on yourself, a crossleg position might be easiest.

- Begin right above the top of the heel on the back of the leg. With the heel of your hand, firmly *compress* the muscle of the calf. Hold for a count of twelve. Release.

- Continue *compressions* all the way up the calf muscle. Keep the same pace.

- Continue the same stroke up both sides of the calf. Keep the same pace.

HAMSTRING PULL

A biggie! One of the most common injuries in any sport due to the great variety of stress on the upper points here. Nearly all lower body power movements include the hamstrings—in stretch, contraction, or for balance—as either prime movers or as accessory muscles.

Because of this continuous action and because of the forward limitation of the knee joint, the hamstring muscles are hard to maintain at full length. Normal usage is so limited in scope that they tighten and shorten faster than other muscle groups. When injury comes here it is highly debilitating and recurrence is a major problem.

Fortunately, hamstring pulls give you a lot of warning. Early or even chronic cases can be protected to a great degree with proper Sportsmassage providing you give them regular, periodic attention.

Telling Where It Comes From

The three pressure points at the buttock fold determine which of the three upper aspects of the muscle is in danger. If a pull has already occurred, the corresponding point—lateral, mid, or medial—will be supersensitive to pressure. The pull occurs from just below the middle of the thigh upward, and the tightened line of muscle can be felt easily.

When the pain is in the lower third of the muscle extending down to the back of the knee, it is the lower attachments that are of major concern. That's a tougher problem, for these attachments do not respond as rapidly to treatment. Also, the risk of recurrence is always higher with an overstretch that takes place at the knee.

What to Do

Direct pressure and crossfiber *friction* are applied to the upper stress points with the thumb. The entire back of the thigh is *compressed* and *kneaded,* with the cramped area gently but firmly grasped and pulled sideways repeatedly.

A thick, heavy spasm line occurs in the upper four or five inches of the muscle—lateral, mid, or medial—depending on where the major stress has occurred. Work this over with first *compressions* and crossfiber *friction* applied with the ends of the fingers.

IMPORTANT: Pressure of all movements must be gentle for the first sequence. After that, you can work to tolerance. The hamstring muscle will not yield to nothingness, but massage movements must not be rough, vigorous, or rapid. Gentle force is what is called for.

In cases involving the lower aspect of the hamstring, the stress points will be found below the knee, particularly on the outer side. It will be extremely painful, and only a fraction of the amount of pressure allowable at the upper attachments can be used here. The tissue is much thinner here, so the penetrating movements of *direct pressure* and crossfiber *friction* must be handled with care.

Finally, light crossfiber *friction* is applied to the tendons as they pass the back of the knee, and light to moderate *compressions* and *kneading* are applied to the cramped area above the knee.

EXERCISE:

No stretching exercises are done at this time. No toe touches, no situps. You can catch up on them later. Restore motion without aggravation. First restore painless walking, jogging, and easy running. Then progress from that point.

Hamstring Pull

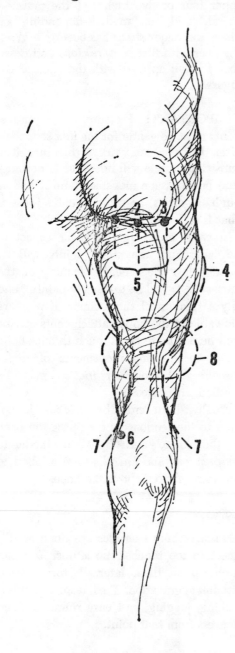

POINT 1, 2, OR 3

- Use your thumb to locate the primary stress point here. It will be very sensitive to pressure.

- Apply *direct pressure* with the thumb. Be gentle. Hold for a count of fifteen. Release.

- Repeat the stroke, still being very careful. Hold for a count of twenty. Release.

- Switch over to crossfiber *friction*. Gently, hold for a count of twenty. Release.

- Repeat the *friction* for a count of twenty-five. Release.

- Apply one more crossfiber *friction*. Count to thirty. Release.

POINT 4

- Begin a series of *compressions* using the flat of your hand. Work slowly and gently, covering the entire back of the thigh. Work down from the buttocks to the knee.

- *Knead* the same entire area, grasping the flesh firmly but gently. Pull it sideways and let it slip out of your fingers slowly and gently.

POINT 5

- Find the thick spasm line extending down about four or five inches from the stress point.

- Apply repeated first *compressions* to the entire area. Be gentle.

- Change to crossfiber *friction*, using the ends of the fingers. Cover the same area, gently, slowly, and thoroughly.

- *Now go back and rework the entire sequence of strokes used thus far*—from the stress points on down. Increase the pressure as you work, but not beyond tolerance.

- Repeat the entire sequence one more time—again, being as firm as possible, but not causing further trauma to the sensitive area.

Point 6

- Find the stress point on the lower extremity of the hamstring—if the pain is there.

- Apply thumb *direct pressure* to the point. Hold for fifteen. Release. You must be even more careful here than on the upper thigh region. Do not overpress.

- Repeat the stroke for a count of twenty. Release.

- Repeat again for a count of twenty-five. Release.

- Apply crossfiber *friction* in the same gentle, careful manner. Hold for a count of twenty. Release.

- Repeat the same gentle *friction* for a count of twenty-five. Release.

- Repeat the *friction* for a count of thirty. Release.

Point 7

- Feel gently with your fingertips where the tendons pass the back of the knee.

- Apply light crossfiber *friction* for a count of twenty. Release.

- Work the same area again, increasing the hold to thirty. Release.

Point 8

- Locate the sensitive, cramped area above the back of the knee.

- Apply light to moderate *compressions* with the heel of the hand. Work it slowly and gently, covering the entire area.

- *Knead* the same area. Work slowly and thoroughly, taking care to give no more pressure than the area can tolerate at one time.

- Repeat the sequences of *compressions* and *kneading* one more time.

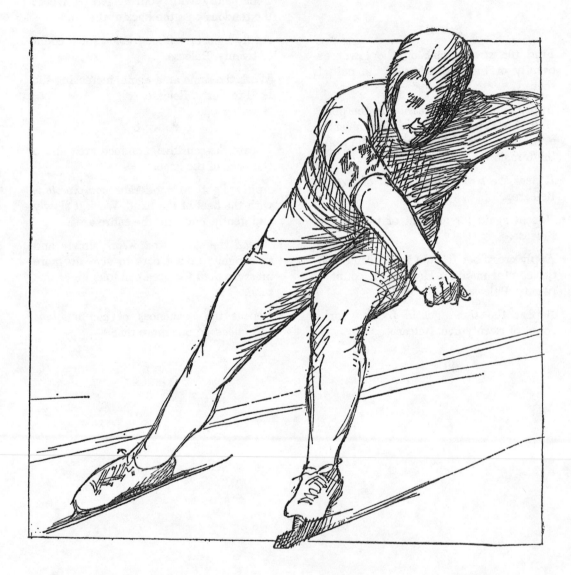

Last year I had an experience that is, too often, typical of the kind of thing that happens a lot in pro sports. The player involved happened to be a hockey star, but he could just as well have been a top competitor in any other major sport.

This happened right before the Stanley Cup playoffs and this fellow was scheduled to play. But he developed a slight groin pull. It wasn't bad, but it was bothering him. Well, what they did was to tape him up and send him out on the ice. This is done a lot in sports—football in particular.

So the fellow made a wrong move and pulled it really badly. When I saw him—he waited a long time before coming and then did so only under top-secret conditions—he hadn't been able to sleep nights for two weeks and he was worried sick about making it to the Stanley Cup playoffs. He was also concerned about having it found out that he had been to see me because the unwritten rule is that you don't go outside of your own circle in sports no matter how rough it gets. Particularly you don't go against the advice of your own trainer and get help elsewhere.

I put him on the table and he couldn't raise his knee two inches off it, even bracing his heel against the table. He was in agony. I saw him Wednesday, Thursday, Friday, and Saturday. Sunday he was skating. And he played in the Stanley Cup playoffs.

But he got in trouble. Somehow word got out that he'd come to me, and they really gave him a hard time of it. Results or no, he had gone outside of the profession, and he paid for it. It makes you wonder in whose interest those kinds of rules are set up.

The Strain of the Game

Hockey, because of the rest time between periods during the game, cannot be considered a maximum-effort sport. But it is an exhausting one, and those rest periods are timed to give you a break whenever you are in danger of falling off your maximum-speed potential.

Yet, as strenuous as the game is, the hockey player—barring injury—can look forward to a lengthier career than can the football or basketball player. First, there is not the constant jarring of the joints of the legs, as there is in a running game. The skates do act as a sort of buffer zone. Also sudden stops and turns are more a matter of shifting weight and balance. And as far as speed is concerned, once you reach full acceleration, you have the force of the glide working for you to help maintain it.

The greatest leg exertion is from full stop zero to one-quarter speed—getting started. After that, the momentum supplies most of the rest of what you need. Leg tightening does not occur as frequently as in other sports where the legs are the prime areas of use.

Contact injuries are the greatest problems, and the effects of these, of course, are legendary for cropping up time and again over the long run. Knees rate high here, as they do with any contact sport, and any secondary lesions that form as a result of knee injuries can be the causes of future problems in any portion of the leg, hip, or lower back.

Sooner or later, that slight forward bend that a hockey player maintains while in motion has to catch up with him. In the older player, trouble here is usually compounded by a host of former injuries that crop up again in a weak moment to remind him of the former abuse his body underwent. Lower back pain is treated extensively in the section on cycling. You might want to look into that.

The shoulder of the stick hand is also a victim of accumulated stress. The popularity of the slap shot vs. the wrist shot adds somewhat to this. It's a good idea for anyone afflicted with shoulder discomfort to check out the three connected areas before a game. These are the trapezius and teres major stress points on the back of the shoulder (these are treated in depth in the section on baseball) and the pectorals on

the chest (see the section on weight lifting). And—a condition peculiar to hockey —stress in the ligament spanning to the top of the shoulder from front to back, which we take up below.

SKATING—SPEED AND FIGURE

It is the legs of speed skaters that first fall victim to that old bugaboo of overtightening. This is because speed skating, in contrast to hockey, *is* a maximum-effort sport. Racers are forced to maintain a bent-forward position that greatly stresses the lower back and buttocks. This posture also aggravates the hip end of the thigh muscles, with the result that power loss and hamstring difficulties often originate here. For treatment of hamstrings, a proverbial problem with skaters, see the corresponding section in the cycling chapter.

Figure skating can be likened to acrobatics on ice skates. It requires a tremendous variety of movements. Trouble can develop anywhere along the line.

Figure skating does not require maximum effort for the simple reason that the length of performance time is not sufficient to bring about an exertion breakdown in the well-conditioned performer. Rather it is a combination of rigorous training and the pressure of competition that are the causative factors in loss of full skating mobility.

An example of training-related injuries came to my attention just a few months ago. Someone referred to me a young skater, well ranked in the New England area, who had been sent to a dance instructor for stretching exercises—a perfectly normal and responsible procedure.

Now, this was a fifteen-year-old boy— very flexible and in excellent condition— who had been skating competitively for years. However, the stretching exercises caused a severe hamstring pull smack in the middle of a standard skating routine he had been performing nearly all of his life.

How come? Because the stretching exercise, even though fundamentally the same movements as those practiced on ice by the skater, put maximum stress where it was unaccustomed. And the boy's muscles reacted by tightening rather than by loosening.

This incident illustrates a rather unusual phenomenon, to be sure. But it is one of those fringe chances that sometimes do happen even in the most careful of cases.

While it would seem most logical that the well-conditioned body would be least likely to be injured in a situation like this, the reverse is often true. The less well-conditioned athlete has a more sluggish response to muscle commands, while the well-conditioned athlete has an instant pickup. And that can put a heavy dose of strain on the muscle attachments. As in the case of the young skater, who, incidentally was able to get back on the ice for the first time in six weeks the day after we had our first session, *the better the condition you are in, the more care you should take when varying from an accustomed routine.*

SHOULDER STRAIN

A shoulder separation—a *tearing* of the acromio-clavicular ligaments—is very painful and severely limits movement of the affected area. If you suspect that you have this condition you should contact a physician immediately. You should never try to treat a shoulder separation by yourself.

A simple *strain* of the superficial acromio-clavicular ligament, on the other hand, is not so painful or restricting. It is not difficult to treat, largely because there are no accompanying muscular complications and the treatment is confined to one small spot.

Direct pressure and crossfiber *friction* are the strokes to use. You begin lightly, then work up pressure to a point that is bearable. About ten minutes total, with rest breaks in between, is usually sufficient to re-establish a normal range of painless motion.

Shoulder Strain

POINT 1

• Have the player sit, stand, or lie face down.

• With the thumb or forefinger, apply very gentle *direct pressure* on the point, just at the crest of the outer tip of the shoulder. Hold it for fifteen seconds. Release.

• Repeat the stroke, holding it slightly longer and applying slightly more pressure. Release.

• Rest for a minute or so and go on with the *direct pressure*. Work for a minute, then rest for another for a total of five minutes. Never apply more pressure than can be comfortably tolerated by the player.

• Change over to crossfiber *friction*. Hold the stroke for fifteen seconds, then release.

• Follow the same pattern and sequence as above for a total of five minutes' massage.

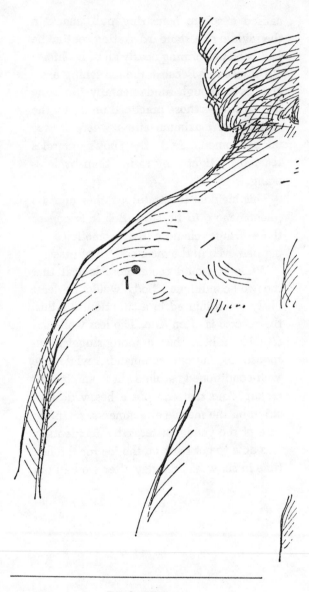

CRAMPED BUTTOCK

This is a condition well known to skaters, particularly those of the figure variety. The stress point is dead center in the middle of the buttock. It is most noticeable when you rise from a seated position.

In order to locate the lesion, you have to probe deep, more so if the person is heavy or muscular. It feels like a very tight muscle mass or, in some cases, like a series of strings. The treatment is *direct pressure* and crossfiber *friction* deeply applied.

In addition, the entire buttock region should be worked over with general Sportsmassage, as described in the Total Massage portion of the "How to Do It" chapter at the beginning of the book.

PRO TIP

A lot of people have trouble relaxing when you get to working around the private areas of the body. Here's a tip I use when I want to detensify the buttock region of a patient I'm massaging: *Have him cross his feet so that the front of the foot of the side you're working on is on top of the other foot.* It's an automatic release posture.

You may have to go back and forth between the general massage and the *direct pressure-friction* routines several times before you get a good response. What is a good response? When the manual pressure you apply is not felt as strongly as it was initially—when the stress point has become desensitized.

EXERCISE:

The order of follow-up exercises for a cramped buttock is: walking, sitting, and rising from a chair. Then full squats with the heels flat on the floor.

The squats are limited at this point—only enough to establish painless motion. Not as a repetitive exercise in themselves. The normal movement of walking, increasing the length of the stride, and climbing up and down stairs will give you just the right range of exercise to produce contractions without any stress.

Cramped Buttock

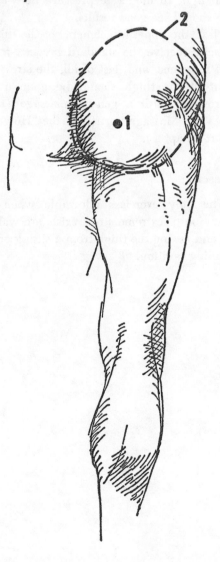

POINT 1

- Have the player lie face down with the legs stretched out straight behind.

- Locate the stress point in the center of the buttock, probing deeply with thumb or braced forefinger. It will feel hard or stringy.

- Apply full *direct pressure* using the point of the thumb, the braced forefinger, or the tips of all four fingers braced with the other hand. Hold for twenty seconds. Release.

- Repeat this stroke three more times. Work as deeply as you can. Increase the hold to a count of thirty gradually.

- Change the stroke to crossfiber *friction*. Stroke up and down the body line, moving your fingers slightly in and out. Hold for a count of twenty. Release.

- Repeat the *friction* three more times. Work as deeply as possible, increasing the holding time to thirty after the first two passes.

POINT 2

- Go on to the buttock general massage described in the "How to Do It" chapter.

- Afterward, you can repeat the *pressure-friction* sequences, alternating with the full-buttock massage as often as necessary to desensitize the stress point.

LEG STRETCH PAIN

If any condition rates as a skater's complaint, it might be this one. It's the sharp, nagging pain that hits you in the sensitive area just inside the front rim of the pelvis, and it comes from skating with your leg stretched out behind you.

Because this position, a perfect example of Basic Movement No. 3, is one of maximum extension, an injury could come at any time. That's why it's a particularly good idea to check out the stress points involved before each and every skating session, especially since the area involved is one of the trickiest to treat after the fact of injury.

Under normal conditions, little or no massage is given to this region because the area lacks surface-muscle coverage and can be very tender if messed with. The muscles involved are the iliacus and the psoas, deep-lying muscles covered over by a crisscross of tendons and ligaments. Any time you feel a preliminary stiffness in the front of the upper thigh, look to this region first as the cause of the problem.

Working It Out

To get at the initial trouble spot, you have to hook your fingers over the top of the iliac crest—rim of the pelvis—and press inward. Or you can get there all the same by pressing straight down with the thumb. *Direct pressure* and crossfiber *friction* are the prescriptions here.

The second point, that of the psoas, is angled a few inches downward from the first. It's too deep to reach with your bare hands, so at this point you should switch over to a *compression* method, using the heel of the hand or the loose fist. Work with light to moderate pressure here and you should see good results.

Next, the upper attachments of the thigh muscles receive the standard *pressure-friction* sequence, and, last of all, the stressed front of the thigh should be gone over thoroughly with a general massage (see the Total Massage portion of the "How to Do It" chapter).

EXERCISE:

The only exercises allowable when a condition of extreme stress exists are walking and flexing the thigh from a sitting or a standing position.

Leg Stretch Pain

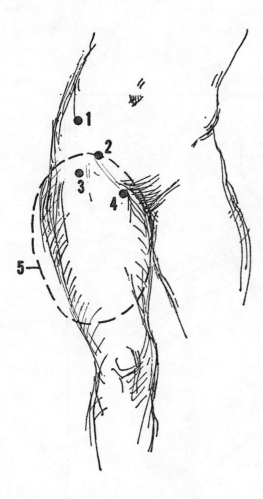

POINT 1

- Have the player lie flat out on the back.

- Using all four fingers or the thumb alone, locate the primary stress point.

- Apply *direct pressure* for a count of fifteen. Release.

- Repeat the stroke. Count to twenty. Release.

- Repeat the stroke. Count to twenty-five. Release.

- Change to crossfiber *friction*. Count to fifteen. Release.

- Repeat the stroke. Count to twenty. Release.

- Finish off with one more *friction*, counting to twenty-five. Release.

POINT 2

- With the heel of your hand or a loose fist, apply a series of *compressions* on the stress point here. Keep the pressure light to moderate depending on the sensitivity of the spot. Work three to four minutes.

POINTS 3 AND 4

- With the thumb or index finger, locate these two stress points on the front of the upper thigh.

- Apply a deep, steady *direct pressure* to each in turn. Hold for a count of twenty. Release.

- Repeat the stroke twice more. Increase the hold to twenty-five, then thirty. Release.

- Apply crossfiber *friction* to the two points in the same manner. Hold for twenty. Then release.

- Repeat for twenty-five, then thirty, releasing after each stroke.

POINT 5

- Apply a general Sportsmassage to the front of the thigh. Work slowly and cover the entire area from upper to lower portions in turn.

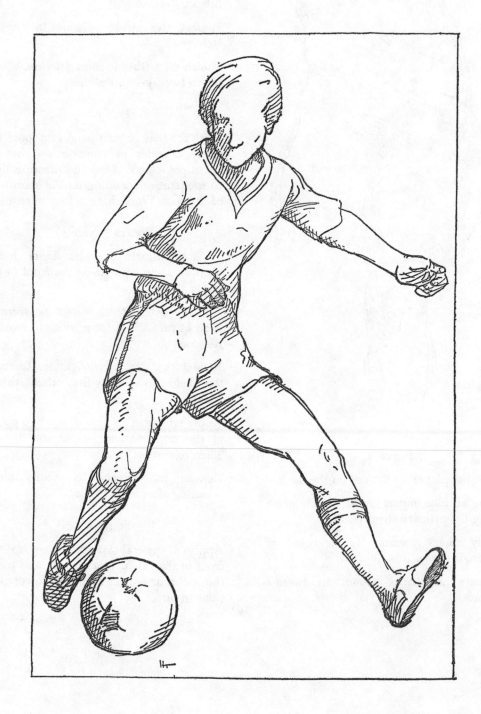

We have a very good semipro soccer team in nearby Peabody comprised mostly of Portuguese and South Americans. Because massage similar to Sportsmassage is practiced in their native countries, many of the players come to me with their problems.

A year ago a fellow came to me suffering from severely strained ligaments in his left knee. This was just before the team was scheduled to do a five-game tour of the Azores and Portugal. We worked on it and the knee responded well to the treatment. The man played all five games without a hint of trouble.

Yet, after the first practice session of this year, he developed a severe ache in the region. It grew progressively worse until it pained him to walk, flex the knee, or even sleep at night. All of the symptoms pointed to a reinjury of the old strain. But here was the puzzle: The crossfiber manipulation that usually works in this situation did not do the trick. It still hurt him to walk, and knee bends were next to impossible.

I had to look farther, and I did turn up an extremely painful lesion against the back of the lower leg just below the knee. Following five minutes of treatment, the player was able to walk and run in place with no pain and to do full squats with only minor discomfort. What amazed me was that the particular lesion that I finally found did not have a direct cause-and-effect relationship to his activities as a soccer player. It was on the left knee, and the fellow was a right-foot kicker!

So I asked him about it and further questioning cleared up the mystery. The man is a baker by trade. During the day he slides pans into a very low oven. And he had been doing this by bending from the waist, keeping his legs very straight. And that was it—the repeated overstretch that was eventually aggravated by the soccer playing! Why it happened when it did, you can't say. Overstretching can catch up with you at any time.

In any case, the player was advised to flex his knees while bending down to the oven. And that was that. A follow-up treatment a week later found the pain completely cleared up, and he hasn't been back since.

Soccer players on the whole are a very well-conditioned group of athletes. The game is physically very demanding. It requires speed, flexibility, and stamina. It also has its share of contact and falls. Balance is an important part of the sport, so that other than falls, the body does not go far off its center of gravity. This reduces the potential for strains in the midtrunk region.

The soccer-style kick does not have the high follow-through that you find in football punting, but it does have much greater stress in the groin area due to the method of backswing used in the sport. Also, other than sprained ankles, the sport lends itself to few foot problems. It might be that the soft playing surface, coupled with the relatively moderate weight of the players, account for this. No. Soccer is a sport that takes its toll from you in the hips, the groin, the entire leg, and the ankles.

KNEE STRESS

The knee is one of the most dramatically correctable areas. Long-standing cases of many months' duration respond to mere minutes of massage. Simple strain here is a most perplexing problem because there are no visible symptoms of swelling, heat, or redness. For all appearances it is completely normal—it bends, it straightens, it walks. But anything more than the slightest flexion hurts like crazy.

The strain causing the problem arises from a twisting movement made with the heel flat on the floor. Flexing the knee causes the greatest stress on both the muscles and the ligaments surrounding the knee joint and so is the most likely pain-producing move you can make when an injury is present.

In simple terms, the ligaments are frozen or stuck. To free them, a combination of *direct pressure* and crossfiber *friction* do a remarkable job. The exact spot of restriction can vary slightly from front to back. Pain is the signal that you have found it.

A three- or four-minute session of Sportsmassage brings a great increase in pain-free movement. Follow this with a test—walking and performing a series of progressively deeper squats—to see how much freedom has been achieved. You can do up to three sequences of strokes at that first session. However, if a full, painless squat can be done after the first or second sequence, *stop*. You have done all that can be done, so don't take a chance on traumatizing an already overworked area.

If the situation recurs in a few days, as can very well happen with long-standing cases, repeat the treatment. It might take a few sessions before the relief becomes permanent.

To get back into an exercise routine, you can start out with muscle setting—tightening the quadriceps of the thighs with the knee held straight. That's about it at first. Repetitive squats should not be done as an exercise until the condition has cleared up completely for a week or two.

Knee Stress

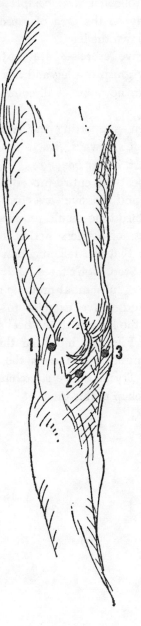

POINT 1, 2, OR 3

- Have the player stretch the sore leg out straight, in as comfortable a position as possible.

- Only *one* of the indicated stress points will be responsible for the discomfort. Find that spot.

- Using your index finger, braced by the middle finger, apply *direct pressure* to the point. Hold for a count of thirty. Release.

- Reapply *pressure*. Hold again for a count of thirty. Keep it deep and steady. Release.

- Apply one more *direct-pressure* stroke for a count of thirty. Release.

- Change over to crossfiber *friction*. Work deeply and evenly for a count of thirty. Release.

- Repeat the stroke, increasing the pressure and length of time slightly. Release.

- Repeat the same stroke once more. Release.

- Repeat the two-stroke sequence—*direct pressure* followed by crossfiber *friction*—twice more. Hold each stroke for a count of thirty to forty-five seconds. Then release.

- After testing out the results of the massage, you can repeat the sequence if necessary, but not more than a total of three sequences should be done at the time.

GROIN PULL

This might be called the grandaddy of all sports-related injuries. It's one of the most painful and, even more unfortunately, one of the most abused conditions that can occur. Basically it is caused by an overstretch in a leg-sideward stretch position, a variation of Basic Movement No. 4. In practically every instance soreness, tightening, and discomfort in motion precede the final strain, the one that makes you think you've suddenly been stabbed by a hot poker.

The first indication of a problem is a deep soreness about three or four inches below the crotch—in the adductor longus, if you want to get technical. Common practice is to tape this and to keep on going. Okay. You are then supporting the muscle to a degree, but you are offering no protection whatever to the danger point at the tendon or origin and are in fact causing even more damage and inflammation to occur there. With enough determination, you can continue to play with these preliminary symptoms, but when a tear finally occurs at the origin, your game is over for good until it's completely healed up!

Higher up and deeper in the inner thigh is the gracilis, a thin slip of muscle that when damaged at its origin causes excruciating pain and makes movement virtually impossible. Sportsmassage here—if you catch it early enough—brings dramatic relief. The gracilis, at the bone and for about three inches down the inside of the thigh, feels like a violin string when it's tight. This is where you have to start to relieve the pressure or nothing you do elsewhere will have any effect.

Work on this point must be very gentle at first, even though it may not feel so gentle to the touch. *Friction* here and on the adductor longus is the first step to recovery, followed by *compressions* applied directly on the area of muscle spasm farther down the leg.

Passive exercises are next. Slowly and gently grasp the leg and flex it at the hip, *just* to the point of discomfort. *Never beyond.*

Then, supporting the straightened leg, move it sideways, *just* to the point of discomfort. *Never beyond.*

Repeat the entire procedure—Sportsmassage and passive exercises—three times. The third time should produce a significant increase of painless motion. If it doesn't, it means that the inflammation has not subsided. Stop. Don't force it.

But if substantial progress occurred, you can add active exercise to the regimen. Bend the knee with the heel sliding up the table. Flex the hip from this fully bent-knee position and cross the leg over the other. Try no active stretching or straight-leg pickup at this time.

Groin Pull

POINT 1

• Have the player lie face up with the legs spread slightly apart—about eight inches at the ankles.

• Lay the pad of the thumb or forefinger against the point for a few seconds.

• Very gently, begin a slow crossfiber *friction*. Keep it up for three or four minutes. Release.

POINT 2

• Move thumb or forefinger forward about an inch. Find the spot and wait a few seconds.

• Very gently, begin a slow crossfiber *friction*. Continue for three or four minutes. Then release.

• Repeat both stroke sequences three or four times gently.

POINT 3

• Move down to the spasm itself—about four to five inches below.

• Using the pads of your fingertips, begin a series of *compressions* to the muscle. Work slowly and carefully for a minute or two. Release.

TURNED ANKLE

The frequency with which this injury occurs reduces its severity in people's minds. Yet the turned or sprained ankle is the most common site of chronic recurrence. A turned ankle is an actual dislocation that relocated itself, rupturing in the process a series of tissues and blood vessels.

When it happens, you should do two things: Get off it; and get it seen to, to determine the extent of the damage. Don't be a hero, no matter how badly you want to finish off the game or series. Soccer is too quick and demanding a sport to have any mercy for someone playing with a debilitated ankle, and you'll only increase tissue damage and internal blood seepage if you push yourself!

Allow a week before applying Sportsmassage. This gives tissues time to mend before you begin massage to restore pliability.

Because the actual location of the ruptures varies from case to case, depending upon the position of the ankle at the time of sprain, there are no definite stress points as such. You have to locate the adhesions by feel. In the beginning, use only enough pressure to barely move the injured tissue. Use crossfiber *friction* below the injury,

giving each tender spot its share of gentle massage.

On the instep, where tendons and ligaments have also been stressed, apply a circular *friction*, then a crossfiber stroke.

A very painful area is found on the outer side of the leg about three inches above the ankle, and this responds well to both *direct pressure* and crossfiber *friction*.

Work on the calf as well. *Compressions* should be done along the entire outside and back of the calf. All of these accessory structures are stressed by a twisted ankle. Failure to relieve the secondary lesions in these areas reduces the amount of motion you recover and leaves you open to the possibility of recurrence.

Turned Ankle

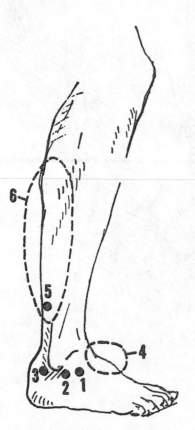

POINTS 1, 2, AND 3

- The player sits with the sore ankle out straight, supported from beneath.

- With thumb or forefinger, apply crossfiber *friction* to these points very gently. Massage each point very lightly for a count of fifteen. Release.

POINT 4

- Place the heel of the hand on the lower instep. Apply gentle *friction*, working upward in slow, circular patterns. Go all the way up to the ankle—sides first, then the middle. Count to ten before moving on to a new spot. Then release.

- Return to the base of the instep. Using the flat of your thumb, apply a slow, steady crossfiber *friction* here. Work for fifteen seconds. Release.

- Move up a little farther. Reapply the *friction*, working up to a count of fifteen. Release.

- Go with the crossfiber *friction*, working on the ligaments and tendons between the bones. Use the same stroke all the way up to the ankle.

POINT 5

- Put the flat of your thumb on the stress point on the outer ankle. Give *direct pressure* for a count of fifteen. Release.

- Repeat the procedure two more times. Take care not to press harder than is comfortable.

- Change to crossfiber *friction.* Hold each stroke for a count of ten, then release.

- Do two more sequences of *friction* at the same pace and timing.

POINT 6

- Have the player lie flat on the stomach with the foot hanging over the edge of the table in a nonhurtful position. For self-massage, try bending down and working on the back of the calf from a seated position.

- Start at the back of the leg right above the upper heel. Use the heel of your hand to firmly *compress* the muscle beneath. Hold for twelve. Release.

- Work all the way up the calf in the same way.

- Then work up either side of the calf using the same *compression* technique.

PRO TIP

Exercise follow-ups for turned ankles are extremely important. Here is the sequence I suggest to the athletes I treat for this problem:

First, a passive exercise applied at the first session. Just straight flexion and extension. No twisting or side bending.

The most important factor is to re-establish *normal* walking as soon as possible. Most people, unless they are told differently, restrict ankle motion while walking long after it is necessary. By doing so, they lose an essential recovery process.

A normal step is one in which weight shifts to the ball of the foot, which gives the final balance and forward propulsion to the toes. When you're "saving" your steps, you loose this final phase and tend to come flat off the foot. You encourage shortened, restricted muscle movement.

The keys to progression are painless weight bearing and normal movement. Until these are present, no side bending should be done. But once it is, you should begin an exercise of rolling onto the outside of the feet to strengthen the ankle area against further sprains.

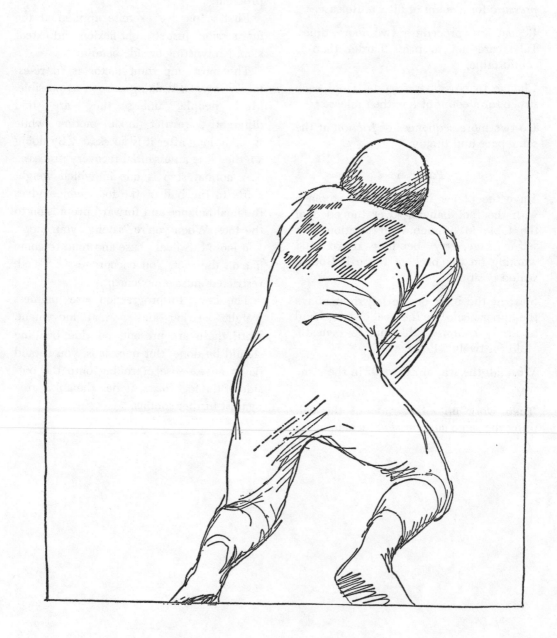

FOOTBALL

The All-American sport is part of the All-American dream. We all like to hear the roar of the crowd and to cheer for our own personal success story. From my viewpoint, when I can get behind somebody like Jim Nance or the thirty-three-year-old rookie and give them that extra boost, that extra chance, that's my piece of the All-American pie.

Football is a rough sport. Any time you have a couple of 240-pound bruisers coming at each other full speed you can expect a lot of fallout injuries along the way. In that sense, it's hard to pick out the problem areas that characterize football. Sometimes they encompass a minute area—such as a thumb strain or a shoulder separation—and sometimes they take over an entire limb or section of the body. As with any heavy-contact sport, a good deal of the usage of Sportsmassage is directed toward repair as well as maintenance. For that reason, in this chapter we will concentrate on a few areas widely spaced throughout the body that represent the kind of stress typical of this rugged sport.

THUMB STRAIN

Probably one of the most frustrating injuries that occurs to a football player is a simple thumb strain. Here is a 250-pound giant all fired up for mayhem and the ball slips away from his grip because a strained thumb simply won't hold onto it!

This is not an uncommon occurrence. Grasping is an inherent part of the game, and the human football machine is no stronger than its weakest link.

In the case of thumb strain, the original strain and therefore the pressure point is in the upper middle of the oval-shaped pad of flesh leading to the thumb. It feels like an unyielding mass line running from the stress point out to the junction of the thumb. Pain is felt in grasping and is not worst at the stress point, but rather in the thumb itself.

The trick is to apply moderate *direct pressure* with either the point of the thumb or a finger directly on the point, holding it for a minute or so. Crossfiber *friction* follows—two to three minutes on the point, then a pass down the length of the spasmed muscle to the thumb.

Go on to treat the entire muscle mass to a series of deep circular *frictions*. Then return to the stress point for some follow-up deep *direct* pressure and crossfiber *friction* strokes.

To exercise the strain without further damage, you can repeatedly press the thumb against the little finger. Do no backward stretching of the thumb for the time being.

Strained Thumb

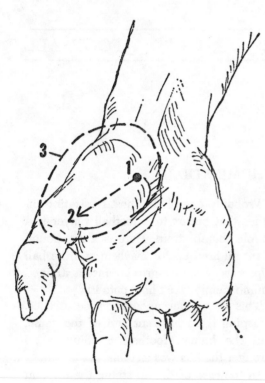

POINT 1

- Have the player hold his hand in a palm-up position, supporting it against something.

- Apply moderate *direct pressure* with the point of the thumb or finger. Hold for a count of twenty. Release.

- Repeat the stroke two more times.

- Change to crossfiber *friction*. Hold for a count of twenty. Release.

- Repeat the *friction*. Hold for a count of thirty. Release.

- Repeat thirty-second passes of crossfiber *friction* for another two minutes, releasing the press between strokes.

POINT 2

- Work on with the crossfiber *friction*, moving down the length of the spasm to the junction with the thumb. Work slowly, using moderate pressure.

POINT 3

- Massage the entire oval of muscle, using deep, circular *friction* applied with the point of the thumb. Go deeply and work steadily.

- Return to the original stress point. Apply deeper *direct pressure* and crossfiber *friction*, holding each stroke for a count of thirty, then releasing. Work for two minutes total.

SHOULDER STRAIN

This injury, a fallout of heavy-contact sports such as football, hockey, or soccer, occurs at the point where the shoulder blade and the collarbone join each other, attached by ligaments. The injury is a tearing or a stretching of these ligaments.

Pain is felt directly in the shoulder joint, sometimes when you move it one way, sometimes when you move it another. Treatment is pretty direct and highly successful.

Begin with light *direct pressure* and crossfiber *friction* and work up to a pressure that is deeper but bearable. It takes about ten minutes—breaking in between—to re-establish a normal range of pain-free motion.

Shoulder Strain

POINT 1

- The player can sit, stand, or lie down.

- Use your thumb or forefinger to apply a very gentle *direct pressure* on the point, just at the outer tip of the shoulder. Hold for a count of fifteen. Release.

- Repeat, holding the stroke for a slightly longer time and increasing the pressure slightly. Release.

- Rest for a minute or so and go on with the *direct pressure*. Work another minute, then rest again. Keep this pattern up for another five minutes. Never apply more pressure than can be comfortably tolerated.

- Switch your stroke to crossfiber *friction*. Hold for a count of fifteen. Release.

- Follow the same pattern as above for a five-minute off-and-on sequence.

LOWER BACK, HAMSTRING STRAIN

Trouble in this area of the body is related to a squatting posture or strain accrued while in that posture. The stress point is right in the middle of the buttock and is most painful when you get up from a sitting position.

To find the trouble spot, you have to get deep into the mass of muscle tissue on the buttock. The spasm feels like a tight ball or perhaps a series of strings. Treat it with *direct pressure* and crossfiber *friction,* working deeply.

After this, go on to a general massage of

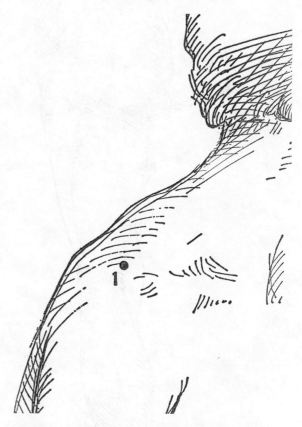

the entire buttock area as described in the Total Massage section at the beginning of the book.

EXERCISE:

After working out on the spot with Sportsmassage, graduate to the following exercises: walking, sitting, and rising from a chair, followed by full squats, keeping the heels flat on the floor.

As far as the squats go, limit them at this point—only as many as are necessary to establish painless movement. Keep them as a general form of exercise until later.

Lower Back, Hamstring Strain

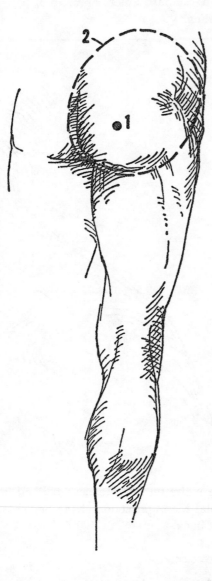

POINT 1

- Have the player lie face down, legs out straight behind. Crossed at the ankle, sore side on top, if especially tense.

- Find the stress point in the center of the buttock, pressing deeply with thumb or braced forefinger. It feels hard or stringy.

- Apply full, deep *direct pressure*, using the point of the thumb, the braced

forefinger, or the tips of all four fingers braced with the other hand. Hold for a count of twenty. Release.

- Repeat the stroke three more times. Work as deeply as possible. Increase the time held to thirty.

- Change the stroke to crossfiber *friction*. Stroke up and down the body line, moving your fingers slightly in and out. Hold each stroke for a count of twenty. Release.

- Repeat the stroke three more times. Work as deeply as possible. Increase the hold to thirty after the first two passes.

POINT 2

- Go on to do a general massage of the entire buttock, described in the Total Massage section.

- You can now repeat the *direct-pressure* and *friction* sequences, alternating with the full-buttock massage until the stress point shows markedly less sensitivity to pressure.

PRO TIP

A tip for young football players working to develop their legs: *Don't overdo the squats.* It will make the quadriceps muscle in the front of the thigh more susceptible to "charley horse" as a result of a blow. It overdevelops.

In particular, I am referring to the use of squats with heavy weights. Any time I work on a man who has done an exceptional job on his body, I want to know how he did it. The most impressive pair of legs I ever worked on—even more so than Jim Nance—belonged to a 250-pound fullback named "Crash" Craddock.

His one and only leg exercise and one that provided tremendous benefits to his entire body as well, was to run up and down stairs with 100-pound sack of dirt on each shoulder. Now, this is an exercise that forces the legs in a completely natural manner. Not only will it build up endurance, but also the leg development is *running* development.

The squat is not natural to running. It is natural to lifting, so what develops as a result of intensive use of this exercise is not a running improvement. Over the years quite a few youngsters who have come to me with thigh problems have changed to this method of leg training with very good results.

It's easy to get the gear for it too. You can find the bags of dirt at any lawn and garden supply store. If you think it's a bit too far-out an idea, you might be interested to know that the same method is used by one of the country's top college coaches, who has his team run up and down the stadium steps carrying a teammate on their backs!

Part Three

This section is intended for use on its own in emergency situations when you need help fast for a particular injury. Arranged according to body structure, each "on the spot" tells you what to do when pain or discomfort occurs in a particular area of the body.

"On the spots" can also be used in conjunction with the sport-specific material included in the individual chapters.

"On the Spot" Sportsmassage Emergency Measures

HAND

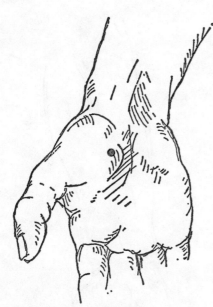

Symptom	Painful motion of thumb at junction.
Cause	Overstretch trauma from thumb bending backward. Overuse from grasping, writing, holding small object for prolonged periods.
Therapy	*Direct pressure,* crossfiber *friction.*

HAND

Symptom	Finger pain.
Cause	Finger bent sideways.
Therapy	*Friction* to joint ligaments.

HAND

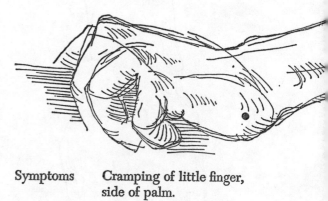

Symptoms	Cramping of little finger, side of palm.
Cause	Overuse strain of little finger.
Therapy	*Direct pressure.*

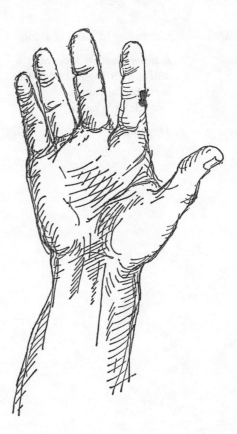

HAND

WRIST (front)

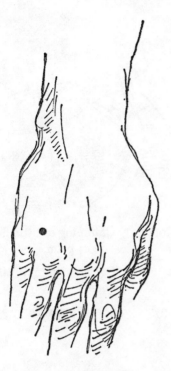

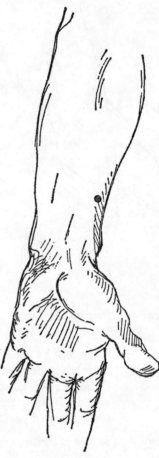

Symptom	Cramping in back of hand.
Cause	A blow, usually a corner surface hitting between the metacarpal bones. "Politician's hand."
Therapy	*Direct pressure.*

Symptom	Pain just above thumb.
Cause	Overstretch or overuse to brachio-radialis at transverse carpal ligament.
Therapy	*Friction* at ligament. *Direct pressure* at muscular-tendonous junction.

WRIST (front)

WRIST (front)

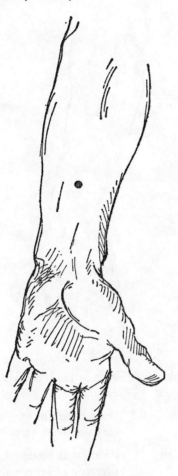

Symptom	Pain in middle of wrist.
Cause	Overstretch or overuse of flexor carpi radialis.
Therapy	*Friction* at ligament. *Direct pressure* to muscular-tendonous junction.

Symptoms	Pain in little finger, side of wrist.
Cause	Overstretch or overuse to flexor carpi ulnaris.
Therapy	*Friction* to ligament. *Direct pressure* at muscular-tendonous junction.

WRIST (back)

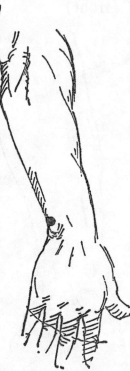

Symptom	Pain in back of wrist on little-finger side.
Cause	Overstretch or overuse of extensor carpi ulnaris.
Therapy	*Friction* at ligament. *Pressure* at junction.

WRIST (back)

Symptom	Pain in back of wrist in middle.
Cause	Overstretch or overuse of common extensors.
Therapy	*Friction* at ligament. *Pressure* at junction.

WRIST (back)

Symptom	Pain in back of wrist on thumb side around bony prominence.
Cause	Overstretch or overuse to extensor carpi radialis.
Therapy	*Direct pressure* to junction. *Friction* to ligament.

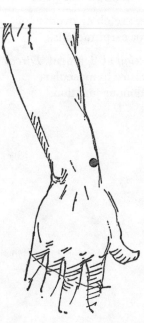

ELBOW

ELBOW

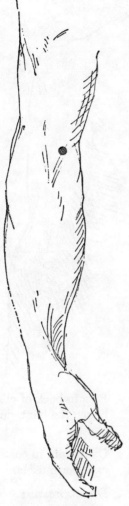

Symptoms	Pain or ache in medial area.
Cause	Forearm strain involving flexor carpi ulnaris.
Therapy	*Friction* applied at medial epicondyle.

Symptoms	Starts as pain in front of elbow. Loss of flexing power develops.
Cause	Overuse or overstretch of biceps brachialis.
Therapy	*Friction* to front of joint. *Direct pressure* and *friction* to muscle belly by squeezing.

ELBOW

ELBOW

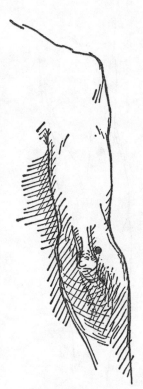

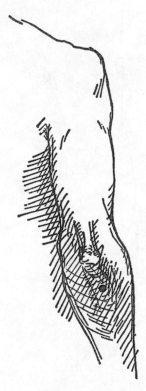

Symptom	Pain in back of elbow while straightening.
Cause	Overstrain of triceps.
Therapy	*Direct pressure* on triceps point.

Symptom	Pain in back of elbow just below the joint, down to hand.
Cause	Overstrain to common extensor muscle.
Therapy	*Direct pressure.*

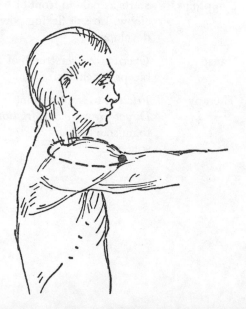

SHOULDER

Symptoms	Aching and pain in upper arm below joint when arm is raised sideways or twisted. May occur on front or back of arm.
Cause	Strain of deltoid at lower attachment at tuberosity.
Therapy	*Friction* to point and length of muscle.

SHOULDER

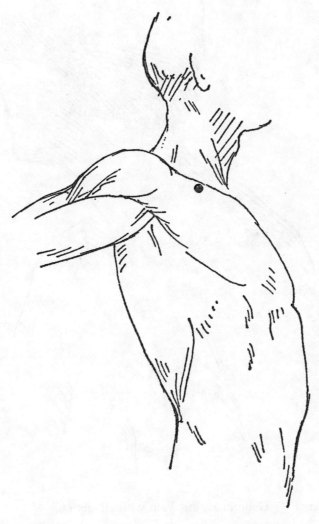

Symptom	Pain while raising arm sideward.
Cause	Backward overstretch to pectoral.
Therapy	*Direct pressure.*

SHOULDER

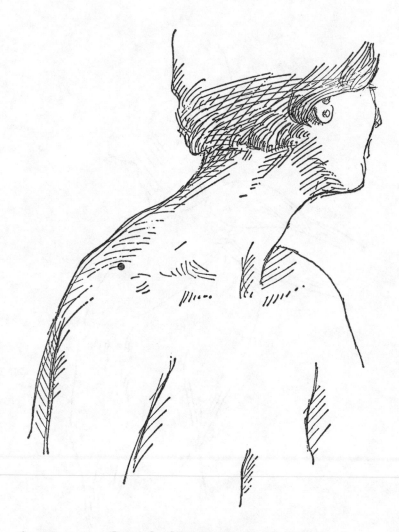

Symptoms	General aching. Pain with all motion.
Cause	Strain to superficial acromio-calvicular ligament.
Therapy	Crossfiber *friction*.

SHOULDER

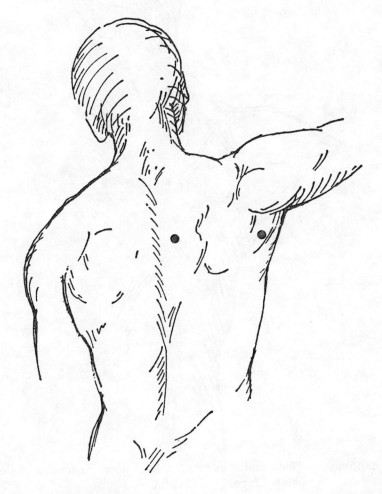

Symptoms	Aching from elbow to hand. Tingling or numbness in the fingers.
Cause	Overstretch to trapezius (mid) and teres major.
Therapy	*Direct pressure,* both points.

SHOULDER

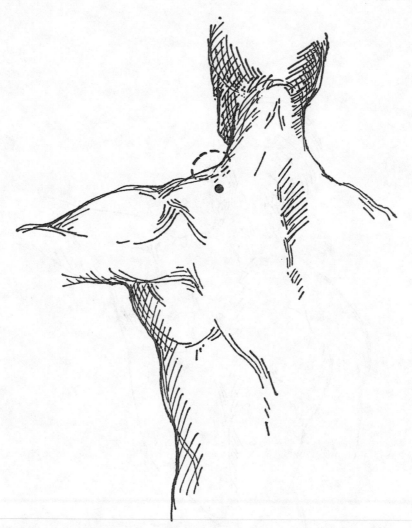

Symptoms	Pain and stiffness on side of neck. Headache on that side. Clogging of nostril.
Cause	Strain to upper trapezius from heavy lifting or from overuse in overhead work.
Therapy	*Direct pressure. Friction* at base of neck.

SHOULDER

SHOULDER

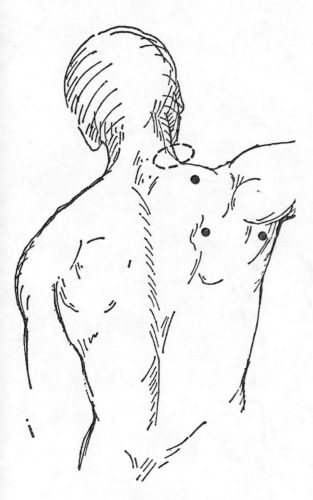

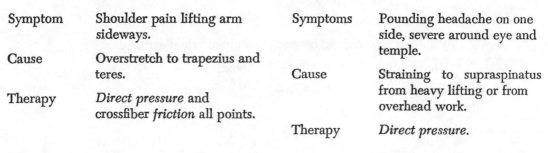

Symptom	Shoulder pain lifting arm sideways.
Cause	Overstretch to trapezius and teres.
Therapy	*Direct pressure* and crossfiber *friction* all points.

Symptoms	Pounding headache on one side, severe around eye and temple.
Cause	Straining to supraspinatus from heavy lifting or from overhead work.
Therapy	*Direct pressure.*

SHOULDER BLADE

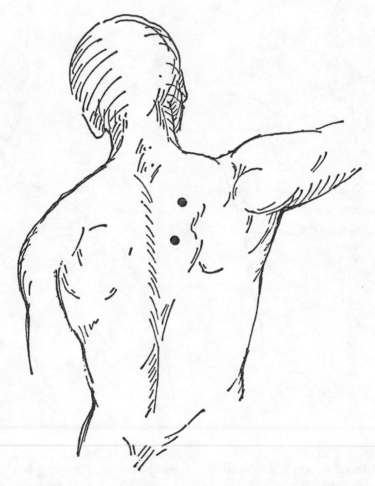

Symptoms	Aching between and around shoulder blade.
Cause	Overstretch to rhomboids.
Therapy	*Direct pressure.*

SHOULDER BLADE

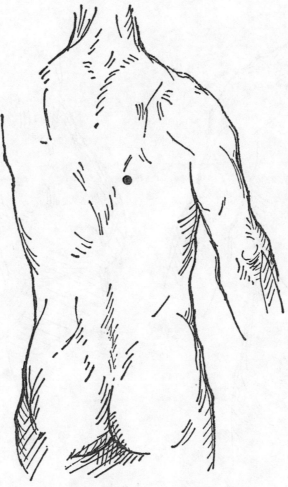

Symptoms	Ache lower shoulder blade referring to front of chest while breathing.
Cause	Overstretch of upper longissimus dorsi.
Therapy	*Direct pressure.*

LOWER BACK

LOWER BACK

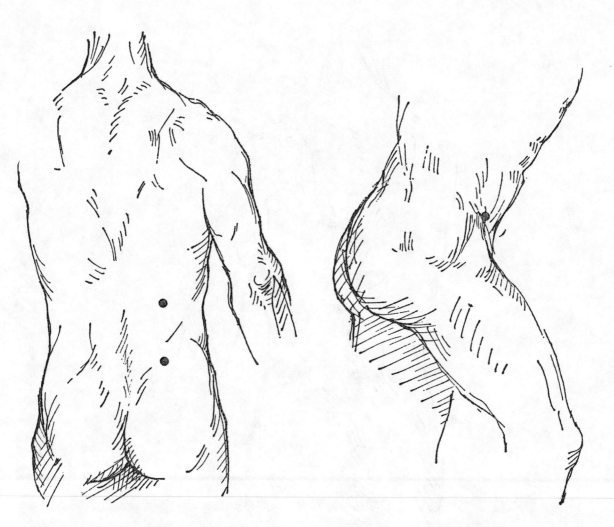

Symptom	Painful forward bend.		Symptoms	Aching lower back and hip. Pain down outside of leg to midcalf.
Cause	Overstretch of sacrospinalis.		Cause	Strain to tensor fascia latae at lateral crest.
Therapy	*Direct pressure.*		Therapy	*Direct pressure.*

LOWER BACK

LOWER BACK

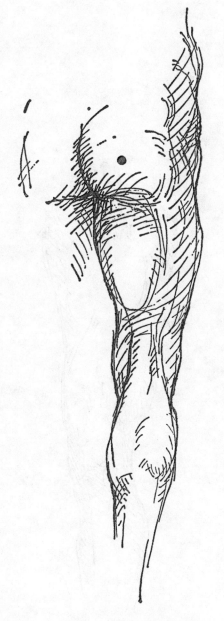

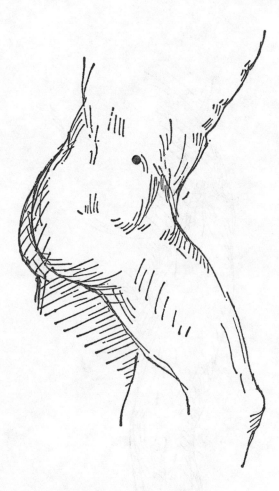

Symptom	Lower back pain.
Cause	Strain to gluteus medius.
Therapy	*Direct pressure* and crossfiber *friction*.

Symptoms	Pain and difficulty arising from seated position.
Cause	Strain to gluteus maximus and piriformia.
Therapy	*Direct pressure.*

LEGS

LEGS

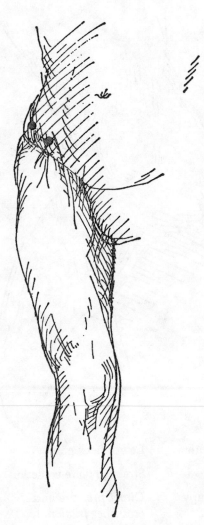

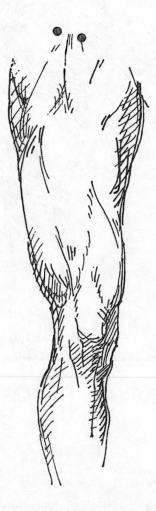

Symptom	Discomfort in front of hip.	Symptom	Cramping of thigh.
Cause	Strain of ilio psoas from backward stretch.	Cause	Strain to upper quadricep fibers at hip level.
Therapy	Crossfiber *friction*.	Therapy	Crossfiber *friction*. *Direct pressure* to cramp.

LEGS

LEGS

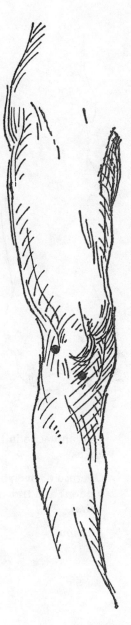

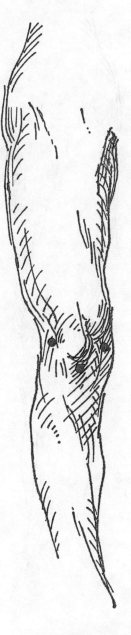

Symptom	Painful flexion while walking.
Cause	Strain to quadriceps expansion.
Therapy	Crossfiber *friction*.

Symptom	Painful flexion of knee.
Cause	Rotation strain either lateral or medial collateral ligaments.
Therapy	Crossfiber *friction*.

LEGS

LEGS

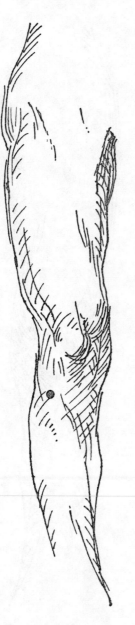

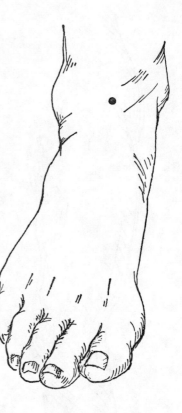

Symptoms	Pain and ache in front of ankle.
Cause	Overuse or overstretch to tendons and transverse crural.
Therapy	*Friction.*

Symptom	Ache down front of calf to outside of foot.
Cause	Strain at origin of tibialis anticus.
Therapy	*Direct pressure.*

LEGS

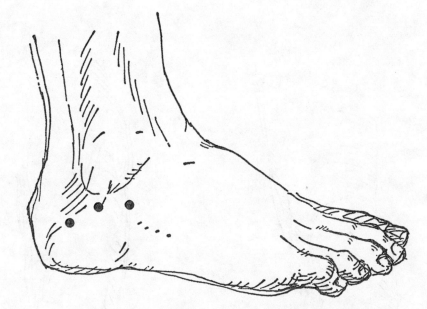

Symptoms	Pain lateral and below ankle bone.
Cause	Overstretch as in turned ankle.
Therapy	*Friction.*

LEGS

Symptom	Cramp between toes.
Cause	Compression to interossei muscles from narrow footwear.
Therapy	*Direct pressure.*

LEGS

Symptom	Cramp in sole of foot.
Cause	Foot in unrelaxed position (plantar flexion) usually following activity.
Therapy	*Direct pressure.*

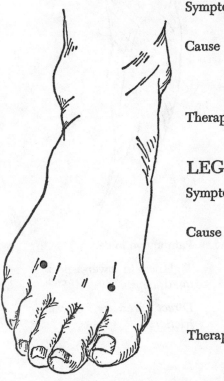

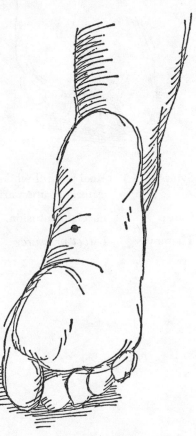

LEGS

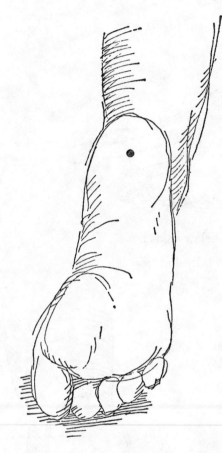

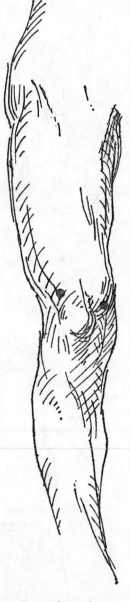

Symptom	Heel painful while walking, especially upon arising.
Cause	Fascial contusion.
Therapy	*Direct pressure.*

Symptom	Pain above knee.
Cause	Tightness in lower-aspect quadriceps.
Therapy	*Direct pressure,* crossfiber *friction.*

LEGS

TRUNK

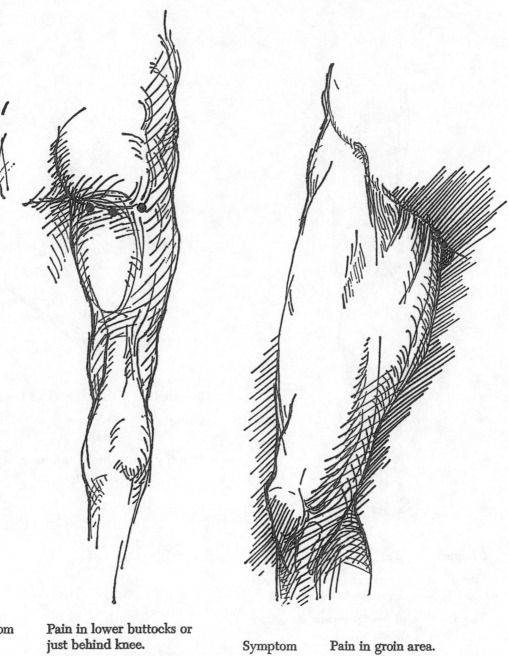

Symptom	Pain in lower buttocks or just behind knee.
Cause	Overstretch of upper or lower hamstring muscles.
Therapy	*Direct pressure*, crossfiber *friction*.

Symptom	Pain in groin area.
Cause	Strain to adductor longus and gracilis.
Therapy	*Friction, compression*. Very gentle.

LEGS

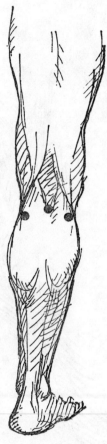

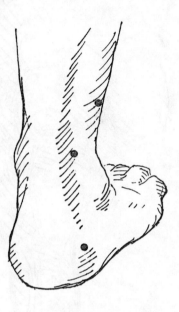

Symptom	Pain in back of heel.
Cause	Overstretch to Achilles tendon.
Therapy	*Direct pressure,* crossfiber *friction.*

Symptom	Pain in calf region.
Cause	Overstrain to upper-, lower-, or midcalf region.
Therapy	*Direct pressure,* crossfiber *friction.*

BACK

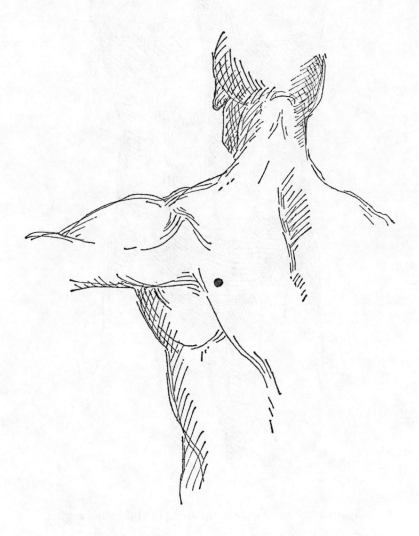

Symptom	Deep ache in shoulder blade.
Cause	Overstretch of lower trapezius.
Therapy	*Direct pressure,* crossfiber *friction.*

ABDOMEN

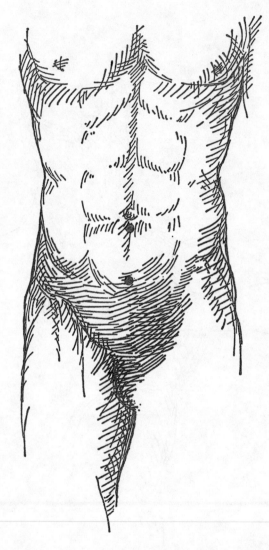

Symptoms	Tension, tightness in abdominal region.
Cause	Spasm in rectus abdominis.
Therapy	*Compression.*

Appendix

FREE MOTION AND MUSCLE FATIGUE

The easier you can do something, the longer you can do it—this is the basic premise of Sportsmassage. Decrease resistance and increase performance.

By reducing the resistance to motion, you reduce a factor of which you are not even aware because you have never been without it. Here then are a few basic facts on muscles and how they are affected by fatigue.

Forty per cent of your body weight is skeletal muscle. Skeletal muscle is made up of numerous fibers, ranging between ten and eighty microns in diameter. In most muscles the fibers extend the entire length of the muscle. In all but 2 per cent of them, each of the fibers has only one nerve ending, located in the middle of the fiber.

Sarcolemma is the cell membrane of the fiber. Each muscle fiber contains several hundred to several thousand myofibrils. The contraction process is accomplished by the fiber folding over on itself.

MUSCLE CONTRACTION

Muscle contraction is dependent on energy supplied by adenosine triphosphate (ATP). The ultimate source of energy for muscle contraction is the oxidation of basic food substances, glucose being the major factor here.

Atrophy is the loss of muscle fibers through disease, injury, disuse, etc. Hypertrophy is enlargement of the muscle. Forceful muscle activity causes this enlargement. It results as individual muscle fibers increase and gain in total numbers of myofibrils as well as in various nutrients and intermediary metabolic substances such as ATP, phosphocreatine, glycogen, etc. Muscular hypertrophy increases both the motive power of the muscle and the nutrient mechanism for maintaining that increase of motive power.

Hypertrophy can occur even though the activity producing it takes only a few minutes a day. This is the reason that strength can be developed in muscles much more rapidly when resistive or isometric exercise is used rather than simple prolonged mild exercise. Essentially, no new myofibrils develop unless the muscle contracts to at least 75 per cent of its maximum tension.

MUSCLE FATIGUE

Prolonged, sharp contraction of the muscle leads to fatigue. It results simply from the inability of the contractile and metabolic processes of the muscle fibers to continue supplying the level of work output. The nerve continues to work normally. Its impulses pass normally through the neuromuscular junction into the fiber itself.

Normal action potential spreads over the fiber, but the contraction becomes weaker because of the depletion of ATP in the fibers. Interruption of blood flow to a contracting muscle leads to almost complete muscle fatigue in a minute or so because of just this loss of nutrient supply.

The percentage of input energy to a muscle (the chemical energy in the nutrients) that can be converted into work is less than 20 to 25 per cent. The rest becomes heat. Sweating is the cooling mechanism by which the body gets rid of this excess heat.

Durable maximum efficiency can be realized only when the muscle contracts at a moderate velocity. Ordinarily, maximum efficiency is developed when the velocity of contraction is about 30 per cent of maximum. Every degree above 30 per cent of velocity, 80 per cent of tensile strength, or the maintained length of tensile contraction as in isometrics increases the depletion rate of ATP and the requirement for oxygen at a magnified rate.

Loss of power occurs when the oxidation of glucose—your main energy supply—cannot take place. The same situation builds up when intense effort or prolonged exertion has used fuel and oxygen faster than they could be supplied. At this point, your body in a manner of speaking shifts its gears into a process called glycolysis.

GLYCOLYSIS

Chemical reactions take place, breaking down glucose—which cannot be converted into energy without oxygen—into pyruvic acid. Pyruvic acid is an alternate source of energy that can be converted into ATP without oxygen. But it is a very inefficient source of energy because only 2 per cent of the energy content of the glucose molecule is utilized in the formation of ATP.

The Law of Mass Action states that as the end products of a chemical reaction build up in the reacting medium, the rate of the reaction approaches zero. In plain words, you have to get rid of the ashes to make room for the coal or the fire goes out. The end products of this glycolytic process—pyruvic acid and hydrogen—cannot be readily discharged.

Were they to stand by themselves and not be carried off, the glycolytic process would come to an abrupt halt and so would you. However, when these two end products reach substantial proportions, they unite with other end products and are converted into lactic acid, and carried off in that form.

Lactic acid is the dispersal agent for end products which would otherwise encumber the process of glycolysis. It is absorbed into the intercellular fluids, finding its way into other cells of less active use, thus spreading fatigue more evenly over a wider body area.

An oxygen debt builds up during the process. You repay it by the heavy breathing you do long after the exertion itself has been completed. When oxygen is once again present in the system, the process reverses itself. Lactic acid reconverts into pyruvic acid, ATP, and glucose.

One of the most efficient muscles for converting lactic acid back into pyruvic acid and using it for energy is the heart muscle. In times of physical stress, it receives large amounts of lactic acid, freshly discharged into the bloodstream from the skeletal muscles.

In summary, the glycolytic process begins with depletion of oxygen and nutrients. The lead-in starts with the very first step you take. The amount of resistance you start with works against you and increases the work load of the contraction process accordingly. This in turn necessitates greater use of energy and oxygen per unit of work. Residual spasms and tightening further increase resistance and lead to faster breakdown in their areas, spreading fatigue more rapidly into adjacent parts of the body.

All resistance factors increase as anoxia develops and the alternate contraction and relaxation process deteriorates. A tense, tight body is constantly using more fuel, even at rest. The release process of Sportsmassage allows the muscle fibers to catch up on their energy supply. Spastic fibers never really catch up.